What We Feed Our Patients

The Journey, the Struggle, the Culture and
How One Unrelenting Chef is Changing
The Way Patients in Hospitals Are Fed

Jim McGrody

iUniverse, Inc.
Bloomington

What We Feed Our Patients

The Journey, the Struggle, the Culture and How One Unrelenting Chef is Changing The Way Patients in Hospitals Are Fed

iUniverse books may be ordered through booksellers or by contacting:

iUniverse
1663 Liberty Drive
Bloomington, IN 47403
www.iuniverse.com
1-800-Authors (1-800-288-4677)

ISBN: 978-1-4502-8565-0 (sc)
ISBN: 978-1-4502-8566-7 (dj)
ISBN: 978-1-4502-8567-4 (e)

Library of Congress Control Number: 2010919127

Printed in the United States of America

iUniverse rev. date: 2/8/2011

What We Feed Our Patients

This book is dedicated to my wonderful wife, Alicia,
and to my mother and father, who have done
more than any son deserves.

Contents

Acknowledgments

I would like to thank the administration at both the University of North Carolina (UNC) Hospitals and Rex Healthcare for going out on a limb and helping us realize our dream.

Special mention to Betsy Thomas, Chad Lefteris, Ryan Conklin, Ryan Miller, Paul Berens, Marlon Davis, Ray and Cheryl D'Ottavio, Lyn Haft, and Angelo Mojica—all still keeping the flame alive. Thanks for all your help in making this real. You guys truly "Get It."

Introduction

Smile on, young restless pilgrims. A brave new world is on the rise.

—Bow Thayer

Over the last twenty-seven years, I have been on a culinary journey across the United States. I have cooked a lot of food and served a lot of people. My quest has always been to try to cook the best food possible with as much love as possible. I try to learn as much as I can from others as I go along. I always want to know more.

I have forever been a student of food. Even as a young kid, I would spend hours watching Julia Child on a black-and-white TV in my bedroom. Julia whacking the head off a fish or talking about *coq au vin* was fascinating to me! I loved it. I had no idea what half the things she was talking about were, but she intrigued me. Her passion and love for cooking set me on a path that I would never regret. I was one of the lucky ones. I knew then that when I grew up, I wanted to be a chef. I wanted to cook.

The reason for this book is that *someone* has to tell this story. Most people would not ever expect or believe the things food service people go through. There are too many surreal and unbelievable moments that happen every day—the people you meet, the things you see, the things you hear. I remember an old Grateful Dead lyric, "If I told you 'bout all that went down, it would burn off both your ears." This phrase in the song "The Deal" was my inspiration years ago to write it all down. We had a saying in those days: "That's gotta go in the book." Well here it is: *the book.*

To many people out there, especially culinary students and chefs working in the restaurant industry, hospital food may sound most unappealing—like a graveyard for old retiring chefs whose knees and backs have finally given out. It may have the stigma of the "lunch lady" with the blue hairnet on her head scooping out canned peas onto a five-compartment tray. It may remind some of a Salisbury steak TV dinner with the cherry cobbler that you had to fold back the tin foil before you put it in the oven. I am here to tell you that those days have changed forever. Hospitals across the country are hiring chefs as fast as they can get them. A *brave new world* is on the rise! And it is exciting to see it happen. Cooks in our hospitals know how to make veal stock. They know how to make pan gravy using the *fond*, or scrapings left in the roasting pan. They know how to properly use a knife. They know terms like *mirepoix,* (aromatics such as carrots, celery, and onions used to enhance stocks, sauces, and gravies.) They know how to properly roast meats, they know how to cost recipes and control waste and most importantly, they know how food is supposed to be cooked. The days of canned peas and three-compartment plates or five-compartment trays are over. The patients have spoken, and hospitals across the country have responded.

When I started writing this book, I was asked by my father, "Who is the book for; who is your audience?" I thought about that question for a long time. Who *is* my audience? Who even cares about this? The answer I came up with was that it applies to everyone because there is something that we all have in common: at some point in our lives, we will all be patients.

This book is for the patient first. It is also for the nurses and doctors. It is for the people who clean the hospital and keep it safe. It is for hospital administrators and it is for the food service workers, cashiers, cooks, managers, dishwashers, and room service attendants who do, at times, a thankless job, but still give it their all every day. This is for those of us who spend fifty to sixty hours a week in a hospital kitchen. This is *our* book, the story of how we all try each and every day to build excellent food and service *one plate at a time.*

Washington, DC, 2002

If you take out the killings, Washington actually has a very, very low crime rate.

—Marion Barry, Mayor of Washington, DC

I had never worked in a hospital before; in fact, I never in a million years would have thought that I ever *would* work in a hospital. Health care was a new environment for me, and I had no idea what to expect. Culinarily, it was so different from what I had trained for my whole life. I wanted to be around good food and people who understood and cared about what they were doing. I was not so sure that was going to happen in health care.

My first job in this new world was in Washington, DC. The hospital I worked at was one of the largest in the city. It had over nine hundred beds and was a teaching hospital full of many challenges. This hospital is part of a huge medical complex in the northeast part of the city. Flanked by three other major medical centers, it is a busy place with hundreds of people coming and going all day long. I had arrived just days before from the sleepy town of Auburn, Alabama. Working in the heart of DC was a huge adjustment for me. Even parking was a formidable task.

My job title was associate director of food and nutrition. My responsibilities involved all of the retail operations in the hospital. This included three cafés, which fed doctors, patients, visitors, and employees. We fed thousands of people every week.

For the previous few years, I had worked at large universities in Arizona and Alabama. I was familiar with large numbers of customers. Nothing was new to me—other than the fact it was a hospital. Serving clinicians, patients, and doctors was far different from serving twenty-year-old college students. However, the change was good. I arrived ready to take on the world and to cook and serve *good food*. Wherever my travels lead me, my belief is the same; my goal is the same: *serve the best food possible.*

I began my career in health care with a fast start. I had to learn the differences between doctors: who were attending doctors; who were residents? Who were the nurses? What is a charge nurse? What does a registered dietitian do? How do you discern the difference between a nurse and anyone else working amidst the major complexities that make up an acute-care, level-one trauma center? What does level one mean? Where is MRI? *What* is MRI? It was all alien to me.

The last time I had been in a hospital was probably at birth. This new world was overwhelming at times. Luckily, I could draw comfort from my wife—she *is* a nurse, and she helped me to understand what everything meant and any other questions I had. She used to laugh at me, especially when I would pronounce something wrong.

There was also the long list of acronyms I had to learn: JCAHO (Joint Commission on the Accreditation of Health Care Organizations), these are the people who survey hospitals to ensure patient safety is being upheld; NPO (Latin for *nothing by mouth*), this pertains to very sick patients or those who have upcoming tests and cannot eat or drink; RDLD (registered dietitian/licensed dietitian); and then all the codes, some of which were matters of life and death: Code Red, Code Blue, Code Walker, Code Silver, Code Grey. What did it all mean? It was so new. Who could keep track of all this? And what was it with all those announcements over the loud speakers?

My previous job at Auburn University in Alabama was a far cry from DC. Auburn is a small college town with very little crime. I lived two miles from work. Now I had to do what millions of Americans do everyday, and that was to commute to work. That first week, I was alone and far from my family, and I was beginning without a clue as to who made up my management team. I had not met with the staff, and other than during the interview, I had never been in this hospital. I was temporarily living in a hotel that I thought was an okay place to stay. Little did I know that it was in the worst part of the city.

The hotel was located at the edge of Washington, DC, right off New York Avenue, close to the Maryland line. I stayed there two nights with the door locked shut. I heard gunshots my first night and thought to myself,

What in the world am I doing here? Was this really a good decision? I had moved around a lot in my life, but I was unsure of this particular move. Looking back now after years of working in DC and getting to know the city, I cannot believe I ever stayed there. That hotel is now boarded up and no longer in business.

In the first conversation I had with my boss, I asked her, "Where can I stay while I look for a home?" I told her where I was staying, and her words still ring clear in my head, "Oh my, we need to get you out of there." I ended up moving to another hotel in College Park, Maryland, next to the University of Maryland, and things got better very quickly

When I first met my staff, they were very leery of me. Apparently, they had seen many managers come and go. They thought for sure that I was just another one coming through with the sole mission of making their day harder. They knew that they had been there long before I got there, and would be there long after I left. Sadly, for the most part, that was a true statement.

The hospital was a union account, which was also new to me, but I soon learned the workings of management in a union environment. It was actually easy to manage, as the collective bargaining agreement lays out all of the rules.

Immediately, I could see the food that was being served in our cafés was in desperate need of attention. I was working for a large contract management company that touted excellent food, but the food was not excellent. It was poorly prepared, poorly presented, and not up to my standards. My goal was to change the quality, service, and presentation of the food, and change it quickly.

The Beginning of the Revolution

If you walk past something you know is wrong and you keep walking, you have just lowered your standards. Never lower your standards.

—Ed Steiner, my first boss in contract management,
who said this to me over nineteen years ago.
Words I try to live by everyday.

It was my fourth day on the job, and I was working in the dining area. We had a busy lunch crowd, and the place was packed. I noticed an elderly woman standing by herself. She looked distraught. She was holding a piece of paper and looking around feverishly. I approached the woman and asked if everything was okay, if there was anything I could do to help.

She explained that she was trying to get in touch with our catering department. She was trying to order a meal for her and her husband, who was a patient. She told me she had called our catering office and that she had left many messages, but no one had yet called her back. I told her I would help and asked what she needed.

She explained that her husband was on a VIP patient floor called Five North West. This floor was a special section of the hospital that patients could get a bed in by paying extra. It was like an exclusive hotel within the hospital. In fact, when you went into these rooms, you almost forgot you were in a hospital. The only reminder was that the persons lying in the beds might be hooked up to medical equipment.

The woman explained they were celebrating their forty-fifth wedding anniversary and that she wanted a special meal prepared. I told her I would take care of everything. I sat down with her to plan the menu. She wanted fresh fish, (tilapia, swordfish, or salmon), and he wanted a rack of lamb. I asked her when she would like the meal served. "Tonight," she replied. I did not want to see her upset anymore; I told her not to worry. The meal would be prepared.

I walked away and said to myself, *"Now where am I going to get fresh seafood and a rack of lamb?"* I was sure that these food items were nowhere to be found in our walk-in refrigerators. However, I had made a promise, and I was going to keep it. I hailed a cab from the front of the hospital. I had been in Washington, DC for only a week, and I knew nothing about the city. I asked the cabbie where I could find fresh seafood and fresh-cut meats. He took me to the Maine Avenue Fish Market on the Potomac.

The Maine Avenue Fish Market is one of the oldest open-air fish markets in the country. It's an amazing place. I picked up a side of salmon, some diver scallops, and some crabmeat. The cab driver then took me to a Farmers' Market in the Foggy Bottom neighborhood. I walked the rows and rows of farmer's carts, picking out the freshest produce I could find. I ended up with some fingerling potatoes and bunches of fresh asparagus, shitake mushrooms, and a couple bulbs of the best looking fennel I had ever seen. Assuming that the hospital would not have fresh herbs, I grabbed some basil, dill, and parsley as well. I made a mental note that I would be back soon to explore more of this incredible produce.

After the farmers' market, I headed to the gourmet store Dean and Deluca on M Street and Wisconsin Avenue in Georgetown. I entered the store and was amazed at what I saw. They had an incredible grab–and-go selection of amazing salads, prepared foods, and desserts. There were aisles of beautifully prepared foods laid out in open-air refrigerators. They had an imported cheese selection that seemed to never end. I watched them slice prosciutto paper-thin to order and lay it out on fresh bagels with arugula. I wanted to do the type of food they were doing!

I was taking a mini culinary tour of DC. This was so much better than Auburn, Alabama, where the only thing you could find in a supermarket were collard greens, potatoes, green peppers, and onions! It was refreshing to see such a vast variety of foods being sold by people who knew what they were talking about and appreciated quality.

Going to this length to satisfy a patient may sound farfetched, but I do it all the time. Going to the store for patients is common. My goal is to please them, and sometimes I just do not have what they need. So I go and get it. I have gone to the store for many items: from gluten-free pasta to Odwalla juices, soy products, and organic produce. I even had a request from a pediatric patient for Skippy Peanut Butter. It was the only peanut butter he would eat. It is all about service, and I am always willing to please. If patients want a certain food and I can reasonably supply it, I do. All I wanted to do that day was help this lady. It seemed like the right thing to do.

The physician upon admission to the hospital prescribes each patient a diet. This is how the kitchen knows what to feed them. This woman's husband was on a heart-healthy cardiac diet. This anniversary dinner meal would not normally be served to him. However, I wanted to liberalize his diet for this special occasion. I went to his floor and talked to the charge nurse. This nurse was in charge of that particular floor. Together, we got permission from the physician to go outside his diet. Both the physician and the charge nurse were happy to make this exception, as it was an important milestone in his life.

I arrived back at the hospital, cooked the meal, and served it. I met the husband, who was a nice guy and very appreciative of his lamb chops, and hung out for a few hours to ensure that they had all they needed. Then I went home.

Two or three weeks went by, and I had moved on to other things. I actually had forgotten about the meal—I have done so many meals over the years that it is sometimes hard to remember what the menu was from any particular one.

I was walking from my office, and I saw the woman again. She was again looking around the room. I approached her, and when I got near, she recognized me. She ran up and gave me a big hug. She began to cry and kissed me on the cheek. She explained that her husband had died and that she was looking to thank me for what I had done. It had been their forty-fifth wedding anniversary, and I had made it special. She said the last days of her husband's life were filled with joy. He had loved the meal and had talked about it till his death. I really did not know what to say. I was saddened by the fact that he had died, but I was happy that I was able to make their last big meal together a memorable one.

Driving home that day, it hit me. I had actually made a difference in someone's life by cooking! I had cooked for many years, working in restaurants, hotels, and colleges, but I never once felt that I had actually made a difference—until this one meal. It was a meal that I had cooked many times before, but this time, it was special. I had made a difference in someone's life. What a feeling that was—and it still is.

I have been cooking for patients ever since that day and hopefully will do so for a long time. This is by far the most rewarding job I have ever had.

The Early Years

Hingham, Massachusetts, 1983

When your name is on the side of the building, you can cook the way you want to cook; until then, you will do it my way.

—My first lesson on following recipes.

I started in the food business when I was in high school. I began where all aspiring cooks start—the pot sink. I worked as a dishwasher at Fiddler's Restaurant in Hingham, Massachusetts. I was sixteen years old.

Hingham is a small upper-middle class town south of Boston. It's located right on the water. I lived in a neighborhood called Crowes Point where my house looked directly across the bay toward Boston. It was a great place to grow up. We had the harbors and beaches at our disposal. Many of my friends had boats, and we would spend countless hours on the ocean. We had an amusement park right on the beach and way too many opportunities to get into trouble. All these fun things cost money, and money was something I didn't have. Given my destitute state, as soon as I was old enough to work, I found my first dishwashing job.

Fiddler's Restaurant was located right across the street from Hingham Harbor. It was a very busy place, not too expensive but trendy for the times. It was especially busy in the summer. The restaurant primarily served seafood, but we also served steaks, chicken, and pasta. It had a very busy bar scene, and the place was hopping most of the time.

As a dishwasher, I was at the lowest rung of the restaurant "food chain." We were always the brunt of jokes and assigned the worst tasks imaginable. It was rough, but I loved both the fast pace and being around the cooks. I thought these guys were amazing.

In between washing pots, I would watch them on the line pumping out three hundred dinners. I was amazed at the sauté station and the flames erupting in the pan as they deglazed with Marsala wine, at the banter between the expediter and the cooks. "Ordering! One shrimp scampi!" "Fire one osso bucco!" or "Picking up! Two Marsalas, medium-rare tenderloin, and a broiled lobster!" I wanted so badly to learn what they were doing. It was fascinating how they could keep track of all that and keep the food coming. It was like a machine.

After a year of washing dishes and constantly bugging the cooks to teach me what they knew, I finally had the nerve to ask the owner if I could move up to a cook's position. He took one look at me and said, "Kid, you are too young; you'll get hurt up there." I told him I would work for free for one week, and if he did not like what I was doing, I would go back to the pots sink. He must have been impressed that I wanted it so bad, because he gave me a chance.

The next day I went up to the line and said, "I'm ready, Chef. Can I work the sauté station?" All the cooks laughed at me and said that I had to pay my dues first. I was not ready to take on the beast. The "beast" was the twelve-burner stove that was without a doubt the most involved station in the restaurant. It was where the seasoned vets worked. They were right; I was not ready for that station.

They sent me to the prep area. They told me all "wannabe cooks" had to start here. I learned how to dice onions, peel potatoes, open Quahogs for chowder, clean squid, de-beard mussels, fillet fish, and stuff lobsters. It was not very glamorous. And I smelled like fish when I went home.

My mother used to make me take my shoes off before I entered the house. I really smelled! It was dirty work. I really wanted to work on the line, but I had to learn the ropes. Little did I know that all of these very basic, but crucial, tasks that I learned in the prep kitchen would help me in the future.

In many commercial kitchens today, onions, peppers, garlic, shallots, and so on are already cut. They come diced, julienned, bias-cut—anything you want, you can get. The problem with all of this pre-cut produce is that the cooks' knife skills suffer; many do not know how to properly dice an onion, never mind *chiffonade* basil. This is especially true in hospitals!

Pre-cut produce was not around in 1983—we did all the cutting. I learned skills that many of today's cooks do not have. It is a different world in today's kitchen. Back then, we did everything from scratch. There was no such thing as pre-processed food. We prepped it, cooked it, and served it.

I worked the prep area for about six months before they let me on the line. I was scared at first, but I eventually got the hang of it. I started on the fry station. This is the easiest—but sometimes busiest—position in a seafood restaurant. I fried shrimp, scallops, beer-battered chicken, calamari, and many of the appetizers that were on the menu. I made salads, fabricated cuts of meats, and basically did anything else the other cooks did not want to do. I became faster and faster on the line, and soon enough, I was able to keep up with the other cooks. They still picked on me, but I knew that they were beginning to trust that they would not have to bail me out anymore when I got in the weeds. I could hold my own, and that, they respected.

The cooks I worked with were much older than me. I was just a kid to them. Those guys worked hard and played hard. I would hang out after work, and they would sneak me beers, and we would sit around in the kitchen and talk about how the night went. I loved being a cook and was becoming one of them.

I remember making my very first hollandaise sauce. One of the cooks I admired taught me how to make it. I was amazed at how the eggs were emulsified in the butter. I was so proud that I knew how to make it. I was making it daily and serving it on just about anything I could get my hands on, even at home. Until my brothers said one night, "Do we have to eat this sauce with everything? This stuff sucks." But I loved that sauce and still do to this day

My brothers were often my guinea pigs in my early years of cooking. I once made a genoise cake, which is a classic Italian sponge cake. I was so proud of it! We all ate it one night, and my little brother, Chris, said, "What is this?" I told him it was a sponge cake. I thought he liked it and was proud that I had done it. His response was, "Is it supposed to taste like a sponge?" I was devastated. I had done something wrong, and it actually did taste like a sponge! I took a lot of hazing from my brothers because of that cake for many years afterwards.

Eventually, I worked all the stations at Fiddlers. When I got to the sauté station, I knew I had *made* it. I could now take on "the beast"! I worked mostly Friday and Saturday nights—I was still in high school—but I could do it. I could have twelve burners of food and keep track of it all. I learned so much in those days. It was amazing to me to put out as much food as we did. I knew then that I wanted to do this for the rest of my life.

Fiddler's was owned and operated by David Wells. He was an aging restaurateur with great knowledge of the business and a very good chef. David's problem was that he was totally spontaneous. He would come up with the craziest things on the spur of the moment. David would often come bursting into the kitchen on a Saturday night with forty pounds of bluefish and say, "Hey, let's run bluefish as a special!"

Because it was usually mid-dinner and we were swamped with tickets—it used to frustrate us. However, he was the boss, so we would make up a "special" real quick in the middle of service, just so he would go away. We always wondered how he suddenly came up with forty pounds of bluefish in the middle of the night. David was quite the character. He was my very first mentor in this business and I learned so much from him. He always treated me very well. I think he saw how much I wanted this and he kept me under his wing. It was not always easy working for him but he was a great teacher and was a kind person at heart.

David was one of many crazy people that I would run into in over twenty-five years of this business. I could write a book just about the people I have met. His craziness became part of me: I loved to watch him work, arguing with vendors, screaming at employees for doing something stupid, or just listening to his totally off-the-wall ideas. My managers today would probably say that I am very much like him. Although screaming at employees kind of went out of the business a long time ago.

My early years prepared me for what was to come. I learned how to be a cook. I learned to sauté, roast, and work the broiler. For those reading this book and who have worked the broiler on a busy Saturday night, you will understand. There is nothing like a six-foot broiler full of steaks, chicken, and burgers. You have to know exactly what is cooking at all times. You become one with the grill. There may be twenty, twenty-five different menu items cooking at one time. At all times, you need to know where it's all going, how each thing is to be cooked, and have some idea when the order will be picked up. It is like being the conductor of an orchestra in some insane play.

Working that broiler became a cornerstone of my future. It involved planning, organization, and above all, understanding the meaning of *mise en place*. This is where you have everything you need to get you through the night—everything in its place. You have to ensure you have all your menu items, garnishes, and back up when you need it. The death of a line cook is when you run out of something and you have to leave the line. It is a fatal blow to the outcome of your night. It also usually involves a severe reprimand by the Chef or the Sous Chef, the second in command.

After Fiddlers restaurant, I moved to New Hampshire to finish my senior year in high school. I enrolled in a culinary program at a vocational/technical high school in Vermont. I spent most of my school days working in a large production kitchen. We had our own restaurant, bakery, and catering department. It was an amazing time. At night, I worked as *the chef* of a restaurant owned by two sisters. I was way over my head. I would read any and every cookbook I could find to come up with daily specials. I really had no idea what I was doing. I was eighteen years old and running a kitchen. I knew after only a few months with them that I needed additional formal training if I were going to be successful.

After graduation, I moved back to the South Shore of Boston and worked for a few months. It was then that I made the biggest decision of my life.

US Army, 1985

It is all mind over matter—I don't mind and you don't matter.

—A drill instructor's kind words of encouragement
as we got off the bus at Fort Leonard Wood, Missouri.

I joined the army in the fall of 1985. I enlisted as a Food Service Specialist. I remember the recruiter asking me, "Are you sure you want to be a cook? The army has many other exciting jobs." I thought about it, but I had always cooked, and I thought this was a safe bet for me. My friends were upset when I enlisted. They asked me, "What in the hell are you thinking?" Why on Earth would I want to leave Massachusetts and go into the army?

I thought about it and came up with a couple of explanations: I was living in a small apartment in Hull, Massachusetts. I had no furniture besides my old bed and a really rotten smelling couch that I had picked up on the side of the road. I had no plates nor did I have any silverware, which was Okay as I never have any food. I went for two months without electricity before I could afford a down-payment deposit on my utility bill. I had shoes that smelled like fish, and I had no real way to wash my clothes. I had a motorcycle and a car—my motorcycle did not run, and my car tags had been suspended by the DMV, so I had to hitchhike to work every day.

My girlfriend at the time was drifting away from me. She was becoming more independent, and we were not as close as we once were. She had friends that I hated, and everything just seemed to be coming to an end.

All I ever did was work. I worked almost every night and slept during the day. Only three months out of high school and I was beginning to think that this new world of adulthood really sucked. There had to be another way.

So, this is how I got the brilliant idea that the army could possibly be a good solution. I was cooking, but I was going nowhere fast. My plan was to join the army and have them pay for me to go to culinary school.

So there I was, forty days later being sworn in at the military processing station in Boston. Soon after, I boarded a plane headed toward Missouri for basic training. I later headed to Georgia for the US Army Jump School (I was a paratrooper as well), and Fort Lee, Virginia, for cooks' school. It was a long journey into an unknown world, with many hardships along the way. I regretted my decision for most of that training year.

Cooks' school was not anything like what I expected. It was the bottom of the barrel as far as the army was concerned. I was surrounded by people who had no idea how to cook and who were not even that interested in it. It was simply a way into the army for them. It was painful.

We cooked very basic stuff, and I was always the first one done. It seemed so easy. We cooked meatloaf, baked chicken, mashed potatoes, rice, and vegetables. I was going crazy; I was bored to death. It was not at all what I wanted to do, and all I could think was, *How the hell am I going to get out of this mess?*

Well, the mess I had gotten myself into would have to be lived out. My three-year enlistment brought me to Fort Bragg, North Carolina, the home of the Airborne. I worked in a consolidated mess, feeding one thousand troopers each meal. That number jumped to around two thousand when our battalion went on alert. The things that I remember most about my days in Ft. Bragg was our attention to food safety, the diversity of those we fed, and feeding those soldiers in an amazingly short amount of time.

Food safety is a big factor in the US Army. We were told that more soldiers had died in the history of the US Army from illness and disease than from bullets, mortars, or bombs. It was crucial for us to maintain an extremely sanitary environment for the troops. Our kitchens were inspected weekly, and we were always at the top of our game.

In the summer of 1987, I was charged with training incoming National Guard units that visited Fort Bragg. I went to the field with the units and observed their ware-washing equipment. This was a critical part of food safety, as the army was still using the mess kit, issued to each soldier. The mess kit was an aluminum dish, along with flatware, that was used by the troops to eat their meals. These kits had to be sanitized each time they used them. The piece of equipment used to sanitize the kits was the Immersion Heater.

The immersion heater was by far the most dangerous piece of equipment I have ever used in food service. It consisted of a tank of gas that dripped into a coiled piece of tubing. The tubing had gasoline combusting at its base, causing heat, which heated the water it was immersed in. The water was in thirty-five-gallon trashcans that were used for washing pots.

The dangerous thing was if you did not start it properly, a fifteen-foot flame would erupt from the tubing, burning everything it touched. It would virtually explode with volatile gasoline. The golden rule was never to put your face over the tubes. I can tell you that I personally burned many a very expensive anti-radar camouflage net that covered our mess tents when I failed to do this right.

The outcome was always a chewing-out and threats of horrible punishment, such as having to pump the port-o-johns—the worst punishment the army could give you. Needless to say, I became very good at my job. I had to do the port-o-johns once, and I vowed to never put myself in that living hell again.

As I have mentioned, food safety was a big part of our lives. We learned how to cook food properly, even though it was not always the best quality. We learned how to make it taste good and look appealing. The food was always safe. We learned about proper cooking and holding temperatures and how to reheat food. This training was vital for me, as my previous culinary experiences had been in a world of cooking where people smoked and did drugs while they worked. This most certainly never happened in army mess halls. We were clean, and the standard was held high by all of those around me.

We had a hard-charging, hard-core boss named SFC (sergeant first class) David Curran. He was an old Vietnam-era soldier who was getting ready to retire. He had been an infantry man years before and got hurt (or so the story went), and they relegated him to the position of mess sergeant. He was relentless in his abuse. He loved to torture us in every way possible. If the kitchen was not perfectly cleaned when our shift ended, we would have to stay for hours cleaning out an oven or other piece of equipment. Every fifteen minutes, he made us stop cooking to thoroughly clean the kitchen. He was impossible. If the food was not right, he would make us do it over. We never served a burnt, undercooked, or bland meal to anyone we fed. That was unacceptable in SFC Curran's mind.

He did, however, make us the best Consolidated Mess on post, and we were always winning awards from division headquarters. We were known around the post as the best place to eat. We became really good at what we did and it was all because SFC Curran never took his eye off what was important. He was a perfectionist in every way, and his unyielding attitude toward being number one rubbed off on all of us.

When I was getting ready to leave the army, he sat me down and asked about my future: what was I going to do with the rest of my life? I told him I was going to enroll at the Culinary Institute of America and learn to be a chef. He was so pleased with me that he publicly announced my intentions to the rest of the cooks. I think he was proud of me and what I had achieved throughout the years. I had been his main cook, and he was often harder on me than the rest. I guess I was his "experiment." In the end, SFC Curran was a pretty good guy who taught all of us a lot about life and how hard it could be. After two years with him, I was ready to take on the greater world of cooking.

Diversity

You will all get along, or I will kill you—all of you.

—Our senior drill instructor with one
of his most memorable "inspirations of the day,"

I was nineteen years old in the fall of 1985. I had lived in Massachusetts and New Hampshire for the last few years. Enrollment in my high school was made up of mostly white students with very few minorities. I had indeed lived a sheltered life.

When I joined the army, there was every walk of life you could imagine. My closest friends in basic training were from Jersey City, New York City, Detroit, and small towns throughout the South. They call America the melting pot of culture—if you have ever been in the service, you know that the true melting pot is our armed forces. I experienced every type of culture from every corner of the country, all rolled up in one band of brothers.

I remember when I was first turned on to rap music. There were these two guys from Detroit free styling in the hallway. At that time, rap was not a mainstream music form as it is today. It could be heard mostly in the big cities; it was certainly not heard on the airwaves of New Hampshire. It was completely alien to me. Even though I was a Grateful Dead fan and loved classic rock-and-roll music, I thought this rap stuff was cool. It was very entertaining, to say the least.

It fascinated me to hear a kid from Oklahoma talking about his farm, then another kid from New York City singing rap music, and then hearing a kid from California talking in some weird, beach lingo that I had only heard in movies. All of these people mesmerized me with the new experiences they gave me.

It was not always harmonious. In the beginning, we all mistrusted each other and many fights occurred among the ranks. Sometimes the kid from Oklahoma would not agree with what the kid from New Jersey had to say, and a fight would break out. But as we slept, ate, and worked side by side every day, we became like brothers. I think we all learned that it did not matter where you came from or what color you were—what mattered is how we looked after each other. In the end, if one of our boys was in trouble, we were all ready to defend him.

Furthermore, living in such a diverse world helped prepare me for the life of a cook. I have had many employees over the years; I have had cooks from Jamaica, Africa, Europe, Asia, and just about every Latin American country. Every one of those cooks taught me so much about their culture and the food that they grew up eating. I learned how to make *masa* for tamales, curried goat and beef patties with coco bread from Jamaica, *papusa* from El Salvador, and many exotic African dishes such as peanut butter soup—a delicious but very spicy soup made with liver, beef, peanut butter, and chilies. I also learned that there is more to life than jalapeños. I was introduced to *guajillo, ancho, serrano, pasilla,* and many other incredible chilies that make up the intense layers of flavors found in these foods.

The most intriguing thing to me was how every culture makes their own version of rice. My wife is from Colombia and understands what good rice is. In fact, she calls bad rice "fake rice" and will not eat it. I have spent the last eight years trying to master cooking rice. It is so complex, and many chefs don't even realize it.

What is the perfect rice? There are so many varieties! And every culture uses them differently in dishes, not to mention that the cooking methods are vastly different. When you come upon good rice, you know it. My brother-in-law's mother was recently visiting my family. She is an older Colombian woman who barely speaks English, but she makes the best rice I have ever had. I have been to some of the best restaurants in America and have never had anything so good. In broken Spanish, I asked her how she did it. She replied, "You need good rice, even better stock, and lots of love." I have never been able to emulate that rice. She is not a chef, but she makes better rice than most chefs working today. She is a master.

I love to talk about the food from other countries. When I talk to the cooks about their home country, I always ask what type of food is served in a traditional meal. I then ask them to teach me how to prepare it. I once had a young Salvadorian cook working for me. I asked her to show me how to make Papusas, which I love. Not only did she show me, she brought in another woman from her community. They came into our kitchen and we made Papusas for 4 hours. We then served these incredible *stuffed masa tortillas* in our café. Our customers loved it! That employee was beaming with pride as we served her country's food. An extra benefit was that the employees soon began to feel that management really cared about who they were and where they came from. The food was delicious. I have since placed many of these ethnic foods onto my menus.

Each culture brings invaluable depth to our society, and I often think about how boring the world would be without the *moles* (pronounced mo-lay) from Mexico, the curries from India, the incredible love that makes up soul food, and the fabulous jerk-chicken from Jamaica. What a sad world we would live in if everyone ate the same foods! I have eaten meals with people from many cultures over the years. And as I ate the food, I began to understand them better.

I think that the leaders of the world should sit down and break bread together. Bread will have different meaning to each leader, but when they experience the undiscovered flavors of a different culture, I believe they would be more civil to each other.

My life was changed the first time I ate turkey *mole.* I tasted flavors I never knew existed and fell in love with Mexico. *Mole has* the most complex layers of flavor that I have ever tasted. I have seen *mole* recipes with twenty-five ingredients or more, from cumin to nuts to allspice, chilies, and chocolate. Try to get an American soccer mom to make that for dinner! I was hooked and wanted to learn more. In the process of learning, I gained lifelong friends I may never have come across had I not shared their food.

I remember spending time in Miami Beach back in the late 1990s and having my first Cuban sandwich at a bar in South Beach. As I was eating it, I could not believe how six simple ingredients could taste so good. This sandwich was the best sandwich I'd ever had in my life. Food is good; food is memorable, good or bad; food defines people and is part of who we are.

Americans are a people of many cultures, and I have always loved to learn from others. We all benefit from a diverse workplace, and I hope to see it become more of the norm and not the exception.

Feeding a Lot of People

It's your world, Sarge; I'm just passing through.

—My favorite saying at nineteen years old

Over the last twenty years, I have listened to my cooks tell me, "We are too busy." I cringe when I hear this because most of the cooks who work in health care have never ever been *really* busy. I guess being busy has a different meaning to different people. In the world of an army cook, now that was truly busy. We had seven to eight cooks cooking meals for one thousand-plus people, and the people we fed were the Airborne Infantry Brigade of the 82nd Airborne Division. These guys were hungry!

They were not nurses picking through salad trying to watch their weight. They were nineteen to twenty-year-old infantry and communication (Signal Corps) soldiers, who were *forever* hungry. The day would start with an early breakfast. When I say early, I mean 0400 hours, which in civilian time is god-awful early or "O-dark-hundred," as we used to say. Thank God for the innocent youth of America. I am not sure I could do that today. The days were long and the work was hard.

I remember putting on my uniform *as* I trudged to work, hoping I had everything where it was supposed to be. I did not care much for the army way of life. I loved being a soldier, and I loved the *idea* of the army, but I did not like the army. There were too many rules, and because of these rules, I was always getting in trouble. I had rebelled against authority my whole life; now I had to do it very quietly and subversively. I would try to create chaos when no one was looking. Sometimes I got away with it; sometimes I did not.

I *was* a good cook, so much of what I did was overlooked. I learned quickly to make friends in high places. A can of coffee well placed into the right hands made my life much easier.

My life changed for the better while on guard duty one night. I was walking my perimeter and I came across a High Mobility Multipurpose Wheeled Vehicle (HMMWV) or Humvee, what civilians call a Hummer, parked in the woods. My job was to report anything suspicious. Given that this vehicle should not have been there, I approached it and rapped on the window with the butt of my rifle. I motioned for the two soldiers to get out. Since I had a radio, I am sure they figured it was easier to deal with me than the sergeant of the guard, because once I called it in they would have been busted. When the door opened, my First Sergeant and a lower enlisted female soldier came out, buttoning up their clothes.

The 1SG looked at me and said, "McGrody, you saw nothing."

I said, "Roger that, Top." I felt like Sgt. Shultz on *Hogan's Heroes:* "I saw nothing …" I walked away and went about my business. I got a lot of "get-out-of-jail-free cards" for that one. He became my new best friend as long as I kept my mouth shut, which I certainly did.

Even with these perks, the life of a soldier is a hard life. I look at the wars today in Iraq and Afghanistan, and I feel for those soldiers. They are all heroes. I was once living that life, and it was hard; we got up early, and we worked well into the night. The hardest part for me was getting up so damn early.

An 0400 breakfast meant that we were there at 0300. We cooked grits, eggs, omelets, bacon, corned beef hash, and the beloved *shit on a shingle*[1] amongst many other menu items. The highlight of the meal was the egg grill—a station that was given to the most reportedly "hung over" person of the day. Can you imagine the job of cooking eggs to order for over 1000 men and women? The sergeants made sure that anyone not toeing the line got that position. As you could guess, that person was usually me. I would report to work at 3:00 AM and begin to crack eggs.

In 1986, there was no such thing as liquid, pasteurized eggs that some food services have available for use today. We had regular shell eggs, which we had to crack. We would crack the eggs into a small bowl and place them on trays. We prepared over five hundred of these small bowls. We would make sure that we had the entire omelet *mise en place* and anything else

1 Creamed ground or chipped beef usually served over white toast.

we needed to get through the meal. There were never more than two of us who would do this. At precisely 0400, the doors would open and we would serve roughly over a thousand troops in the course of three hours. It was a madhouse, and this happened every morning.

Contrary to popular belief, army food is quite good. Every soldier on my watch got a fresh-cooked egg. We would call down the line twenty to thirty people at a time and get their eggs on the grill. We cooked scrambled, over-easy, fried-hard, and of course, any type of omelet they wanted. It was not the army cooking you saw on *M.A.S.H.* Remember, we had David Curran looking over our shoulder every moment. We were *good*. We could get these guys through at an incredible pace. I was an egg-cooking fool.

Today, when I hear a hospital cook on a tray line talking about how there is no way we can do omelets for three hundred people, I think of those days and say, "We did it for a thousand hungry soldiers. It can be done." In fact, we did it usually with two really hung-over cooks!

The biggest and most shameful thing most hospital cooks do is to cook their eggs ahead of time, hold them in hot boxes, and then serve them as needed. The eggs are hard; they become the shape of the pan, and in my opinion, inedible. It is time for a revolution! We can cook eggs fresh and make them edible. I have seen it done before.

Sometime in 1987, the army had the brilliant idea of *not* cooking anymore over-easy eggs. Someone somewhere had done a study and found that salmonella was present on eggshells and could infect a soldier with food-borne illness. Our instructions were to cook all eggs thoroughly. We could no longer do over-easy, sunny-side up, or over-medium. I was okay with this (raw egg albumin is repulsive) and was glad the change was made.

One day I was cooking eggs, as usual, and a command sergeant major (CSM) came though the line and asked for an over-easy egg. I politely told the CSM that we could no longer cook over-easy eggs. He quietly told me that he would put *me* on the grill if I did not put *his eggs* on the grill. He then informed me that he had more time in the chow line than I had in the army and if I didn't cook his eggs the way he wanted he would make my life a living hell.

A CSM is a powerful rank in the army; he is the top dog, so to speak. I was just a PFC, and I wanted no trouble. I assured him that whatever he wanted, I would do it. He probably would not have put me on the grill, but he definitely would have remembered me, and I had learned that in the army, it was all about who you knew and what angle you could have on them. If they outranked you and they had an issue with you, you were screwed. I knew that and did not want to be on his bad side. I cooked his eggs over-easy and wished him a wonderful day. He just scowled at me and moved on.

I never enforced that policy again. If they wanted a raw egg, they got it. The army disbanded this movement eventually, as well. It is hard to tell an old soldier that things have changed. These guys were hard-core and no young punk was going to tell them what they were going to eat, regulations or not.

The Culinary Institute of America

In spite of food fads, fitness programs, and health care. We must never lose sight of a beautifully conceived meal.

—Julia Child

In the early part of 1989, I entered the Culinary Institute of America (CIA). The CIA is located in Hyde Park, New York, approximately two hours north of Manhattan on the Hudson River. It has a beautiful campus and is one of the most renowned cooking schools in the world. I arrived ready to take on the world, to become a world-famous chef, and to make lots of money. In 1989, there was no Food Network or revolving cadre of celebrity chefs, as there are today. But if there had been, I would have wanted that too.

I learned very quickly that the rise of a cook into *chefdom* does not happen that quickly. It was going to take a lot of work. There were some incredible cooks out there who knew much more about food than I did.

The chef instructors at the CIA are the best of the best. They are an inspiration to all the students. The school taught us the fundamentals of classical cuisine. We learned culinary math, meat butchering, and the basics—knife skills, sautéing, roasting, braising, and so on. The CIA also introduced us to the world of pastries, artisan bread making, *charcuterie*, and high-end restaurant service.

The CIA had four restaurants open to the public at that time: The Escoffier Room, Ristorante Caterina de' Medici, American Bounty, and St.

Andrew's Café. The Escoffier taught classical French cuisine with tableside service. The Caterina was about Italian food, and the Bounty focused on traditional and modern American cuisine.

St. Andrew's Café was new to the school when I arrived (or at least the building was new). It was a restaurant based on healthy cooking. That part of the curriculum was called Restaurant Row, the last four blocks of the program. St. Andrew's was the first restaurant on the block.

Before the class started, I was very hesitant. I asked myself, "Who eats healthy food?" I had not done very much healthy cooking, having worked in restaurants where healthy food was not a top priority. It was also 1990, and while "California cuisine" had made inroads into the American palate, in general, healthy food, sustainable farms, local produce, free-range chicken, and organic foods were not as readily available as they are today. I pondered over the thought of who would want to eat food without salt or fat? This was how naive I was; I had no knowledge of how to bring flavor to food without salt or fat. But I was ready to learn. I figured St. Andrew's was sure to be a challenge for me: *Now I am going to have to eat rabbit food. This cannot be good.*

I could not have been more wrong. We had been taught about *roux*, heavy cream sauces, hollandaise sauces, and "barding" our meats[2] with fat for the last year and a half. Now the chef was telling us, "It's good that you learned the classics, but I am here to tell you that the days of serving hollandaise, heavy sauces, fatty meats, and butter-sogged vegetables are over." In St Andrew's, we were introduced to an incredible new wave of cooking that was emerging in America. We were going to learn how to *reduce* sauces instead of adding roux[3], and to substitute vegetable stock for a portion of the oil when making vinaigrettes. We learned how to emphasize flavor with fresh herbs, marinades, and pairing certain foods together to bring out the most intense flavor. We also learned that a good kitchen does not need a deep fat fryer. Steaming, grilling, and poaching were much healthier alternatives for preparing food.

It was amazing to experience how good this food was. We did dishes like pan-seared scallops with saffron rice, roasted saddle of rabbit with wild mushrooms and natural *jus*, chicken roulade stuffed with chicken forcemeat[4] and fresh herbs and then served with a red bell-pepper *coulis*.

---

2 To dress meat for cooking with strips of fat.

3 A cooked mixture of flour and fat used as a thickening agent in sauces and gravy.

4 A mixture of ground lean meat, emulsified with fat

It tasted excellent. It was startling to me how you could make great food without tons of salt and fat!

I remember eating something as simple as polenta at St. Andrew's. Polenta was something I had cooked many times, and is naturally low in fat, so it fit in well with St Andrew's menus. The trick was to make it taste good without too much salt. Ours was prepared and then cooled. It was then cut into shapes and grilled over mesquite wood, with a small amount of pepper-jack cheese. It was so good I can still remember it after all these years.

St. Andrew's training would play an integral role in my development of recipes for hospitals. For many years after the CIA, I cooked food without much thought of salt or fat. I did not think much about diabetes or how carbohydrates convert to sugar and throw blood-sugar levels into a tailspin. The one thing I did remember was food that was healthy for you did not mean it had to taste horrible. You could actually make food taste good without an excess of sodium or fat. It was the beginning of my food revolution, and I did not even know it.

Contract Management

Washington, DC, 2002
Food is our common ground, a universal experience.

—James Beard,

I had spent the last 12 years cooking all around the country. I spent 5 years running a college food service in Arizona; I worked in a 4-star hotel in Newport Beach, California. I even worked in a bank's corporate dining room, feeding people with way too much money and time on their hands. After a few years as the Executive Chef at Auburn University in Alabama, I felt that I wanted to do something different. College food was not fun anymore and I wanted a bigger challenge. I pointed my truck north on Interstate 85 and my destiny led me to Washington, DC. There I met challenges I could have never dreamed of.

I had been hired by a large, management contract company to run the retail cafés throughout the hospital complex. Given my new responsibilities, I was not very involved in patient food … at first. We had a very busy café that took up most of my time. My job was to make money for the company. We did many new and exciting things for our customers. Our food was just as good as any food of its kind in DC. We did Asian stir-fry with fresh ingredients, grilled panini, gourmet pizzas, stromboli, and calzones. We served fresh-carved turkey breast, homemade dressing, and steamed fresh vegetables. We served good food—freshly made and properly cooked. It was not that way when I arrived, but after a year of hard training and setting expectations with our staff, we created a great place. Sales were way up, and everyone was happy—except for our patients.

The patient food that a contractor produces for its customers is often made with very little culinary emphasis. Many operators will use the cheapest ingredients they can purchase and will offer very few options for the patient. This is done to keep the costs down and make the operation profitable. The result is bland, institutional food that gives hospital food its bad reputation

When I say this, I do not mean that they do not care about the quality of the food they serve. They do. However, what I saw were great retail initiatives with heavy focus on the *retail look* and strong marketing tools put in place, all of which played a part in our sales growth out front, very little emphasis was being placed on the quality of the patient food. The money that is generated in the cafés belongs to the contract companies. This is usually the case. When they write the contract, they know they make very little if anything off the patient food. The sales that are generated in the retail areas are where most of their profit comes from, hence the strong focus on making it more successful. Of course, there are many expenses to pay, but it is always the backbone of any hospital contract. Cash flow is important, and we had plenty of cash flowing. Whenever a regional chef or district-level person would visit, the emphasis was always on retail—sales. We had many meetings and discussions on how to grow sales in our retail operation, but I don't remember one discussion about making better food for the patients. It was always about the dollar, never about the patient. This bothered me. However, I did love to create new and exciting menu items for our cafés. I did it all the time. We had good, trendy food that brought great profits to our company.

Profit is not a dirty word; it is what is expected. A company that is "for profit" must make a profit. There are budgets and forecasts that must be met. It is essential for shareholders to see growth of a well-managed company. Making a profit helps fund our raises and bonuses; it allows companies to buy new equipment; it gives our employees better tools and provides long-term visionary growth. Without profit, none of this would occur, and I am very aware of that.

However, this does not mean we have to cook sub-standard food to our patients, and let's face it, that is what we were doing. Our focus was on our retail customers and not on our patients. We looked at patient food as the *other* reason we were there.

The company I worked for did care about the patients *as individuals*. They promoted service recovery, they applauded our employees who went above and beyond, and they had a team of highly dedicated managers whose job was to ensure patient satisfaction.

Our president was an energetic guy who truly cared about what he did. His energy trickled down throughout the organization. Everyone in our organization wanted our patients to be happy and well cared for. We would all visit patients on a daily basis to make their stays as pleasant as possible. However, when selling food for a living, it should come down to one thing—the food. *No matter how much you talk to your patients about how good your food is you're going to have a hard time convincing them if it's not.*

Our goal was to get them to score us highly on the patient survey that would be sent to them after their discharge. Our service recovery was executed with this survey in mind. But almost all of our complaints came down to two things: The "food was bad" and "I did not get what I ordered." It was killing us in our patient satisfaction scores. No matter how many times we went to visit the patient, we could not make the food better by talking about it. My thought was that if we fixed the food, we would not have to do as much service recovery as we were doing. It seemed to me that we were being reactive rather than proactive.

The food was safe and acceptable by the standards in the industry of hospital food. Yet, I wanted it to be better. I wanted to serve restaurant-quality food. I wanted the patients to say that the food was as good as any restaurant in town. I wanted to change the stereotype we were cursed with.

In the late 70s, there was a popular commercial. It showed a Native American in traditional dress canoeing down a river full of trash and debris. The camera panned across the scene and showed all the pollution that had accumulated on the banks of the river. The camera then panned on the man who was canoeing. It showed a tear running down his face. He represented what was good in the world, and the pollution and trash represented what was becoming of the land he loved. It was a powerful commercial that showed us that we should take care of Mother Earth and have some pride and love for our surroundings.

I was like that man the first time I saw patient food being served. I had been trained on quality food; I had worked with great chefs who had an unbelievable passion for food, and we were serving this? I had the proverbial tear in my eye when I saw this food. It was so much different than what we were serving our retail customers. I remember saying that *this* is why hospital food has such a bad reputation. I decided then and there that if I were to be involved with this type of food service, I needed to institute change and bring the same passion and dedication we brought in our retail operations to our patients.

I first had to understand it. I had never done hospital food before, and I thought, *Well, maybe I'm missing something. Maybe the patients are too sick to eat rich food. Maybe they don't want it. Maybe there is some reason for this.* There had to be; no one would purposely produce this kind of food. I began to dig in to get information.

Cook/Chill

Bad food is made without pride, by cooks who have no pride, and no love.

—Anthony Bourdain

All of our patient food came from Baltimore, forty-five miles away. It was produced in a large, commissary kitchen that prepared food for many hospitals in the Baltimore/Washington area. The food came pre-plated in refrigerated trucks. These plates would later be heated and then served. It was awful in every aspect. There were no redeeming qualities anywhere in this food. It was food without love, and that was sad to me.

I remember we were having problems with our scrambled eggs. Seems ridiculous doesn't it? The president of the hospital had received many complaints about them. A nurse who had had enough complaints from her patients actually brought him a tray of food and told him to eat it. He did, and within minutes, he was on the phone with our director. He said the eggs were horrible, and we needed to fix them. In fact, he said it was the worst thing he ever ate.

We had the director/chef from the commissary come down to our hospital to "teach" us how to cook scrambled eggs. The eggs came in sealed bags, which we submerged in boiling water. He said that we needed to take the eggs out of the water frequently and "knead them" like bread dough. This would prevent the eggs from becoming the shape of the bag. We would cook them and then shock them in ice water until they cooled. This was all done the day before they were served.

The next day, we would take cold, cooked eggs, put them on a *retherm* plate (a system with a built-in reheating mechanism), reheat them, and then serve them. I raised my hand during this ridiculous demonstration and said, "Why don't we just cook them as we need them during service? Serve them hot, creamy, and curdy, as they should be. Why are we doing all of this?" The looks I got could have killed me. I could not believe that we were doing all of these absurd things just to serve eggs. Of course, they were horrible—they came from a bag, were boiled in water, cooled and stored for twelve hours and then reheated on a plate the next morning. It was unbelievable to me. How on earth did anyone think this was a good idea?

Eggs were just the beginning. Unlike the café food, which we prepared fresh, we received all of our patient food from the commissary. Some was in bulk form, such as cheese sauce, pot roasts, soups, and chili. I remember serving Italian wedding soup, which traditionally has spinach, meatballs, and pasta. It is really a good soup when done right. Ours from the commissary was made with pre-formed, pre-cooked sausage balls, instead of meatballs. It was not the type of sausage that anyone who cared about food would put on a pizza. We called them rabbit turds. This topping is used extensively in hospital food service. I refused to use them on our pizzas—they looked bad, tasted bad, and were not what the traditional recipe called for. I most certainly would have never put them in a soup.

We had grilled chicken breast that was not grilled; it was put on sheet pans and baked in the oven until a pale, dried-out product emerged. I remember calling the chef at the commissary and asking him, "What is grilled about the grilled chicken? It is baked and dried out." His response was that there was no way we could grill hundreds of chicken breasts for all of the patients we serve. My reply was, "I have a broiler, and I will do them myself." Of course, this was not acceptable, as we were required to purchase all of our food from them.

The sautéed vegetables were not sautéed. They were frozen vegetables that were placed in a steamer, cooked, and cooled. The result was a lifeless vegetable, with no color, texture, or taste. They did not even put seasoning in the food. It was bland, designed to spread across the variety of diets with little financial impact to the operation.

The food that we received from the commissary came in two forms: pre-plated—sorted by specific diets—and bulk. The bulk foods came in two to three-gallon plastic bags that were stapled shut. The food ranged from grits (grits, can you believe it?) to soups, pot roast, and roast beef.

These bags were then stored in our walk-ins until needed. They had a twenty- to thirty-day shelf life.

When needed, the bags were placed in boiling water until the proper temperature was reached. I could never get over the fact that we were doing this. I did understand the concept—it was safe food that could reduce labor throughout the system. As the food was already cooked, you needed fewer cooks in the units to prepare the menu.

However, in reducing labor, we severely reduced the quality of food. The way this food was prepared was not the way I wanted to cook. I was almost ashamed of it. The funny thing was that senior management was always wondering why our patient satisfaction scores never went up. The answer was clear: it was all in the bag.

The food was very safe. It was produced and cooked to the proper temperatures, and then cooled in equipment that would bring the food through the danger zone very quickly. The danger zone is the range of temperatures that allow bacteria to reproduce to unsafe levels. The current danger zone, according to the FDA food code for holding food, is 41–135 degrees Fahrenheit. This means that any food held within this range is ideal for bacterial growth. The idea is to get the food down to 41 degrees as quickly as possible. This decreases the likelihood of a dangerous pathogen contaminating the food.

The food code requires that any hot food be brought down to 70 degrees within the first two hours. Then it must reach below 41 degrees within the next four hours—for a total of six hours. Food that is not cooled within these parameters could essentially be unsafe to eat. Of course, being at a hospital with many people who are already sick, unsafe food becomes even more of an issue than it would be at a regular restaurant.

The food that was cooked in the commissary kitchens was cooked properly according to regulatory standards and then placed into the bags. The equipment the food was cooked in would process the food though a pipe that was attached to a bagging machine. The food would go into the bags and then get sealed shut. Once all the bags were filled, they would be placed in what looked like a huge washing machine. It would tumble the bags like laundry in super-chilled water. The temperatures were recorded on a graph to ensure that the food was cooled quickly. I had never seen anything like it, and it was amazing to watch. I could not believe that food was treated this way. Once the bags were cooled, they were stored and ready for distribution.

The most amazing thing was what they called roast beef. They took raw top rounds of beef, trimmed them, and then put them in the bags. They added salt, pepper, garlic, and the worst thing ever found in any kitchen—"kitchen coloring." This stuff is a concoction of who knows what. It is a brown liquid that adds color to the product. It is an abomination of all that is good. Instead of roasting the meat to get good color—allowing the meat to brown through what is called the Maillard Reaction, the science explaining why meats, breads, dark beer, chocolate, and coffee beans brown when subjected to heat—it was just plain boiled. Instead of using the wonderful pan drippings accumulated in the pan, which could be turned into a savory gravy, *au jus*, or *jus lie*, the cooks bypassed the basics of roasting and used a bottled, coloring agent. It was absolutely against everything I had ever been taught.

Once the beef was seasoned and ready for cooking, it was then sealed by a stapling machine and placed in a huge water tank. This tank could hold over three hundred pounds of beef. The beef was placed on multiple racks. You pressed a button, and the cooking process began. The tank filled with water and heated. The beef cooked in the bags until it reached the pre-selected temperature. It would take about five to six hours. Then, all the water was drained and super-chilled water introduced. The cold water cooled the "roasts" and brought it down below 41 degrees.

The result was what you would expect. Yes, it was cooked. Yes, it was safe—but it was not roast beef. It was a pale piece of meat that had no flavor. It was not what it should be. We took a beautiful piece of meat, added brown food coloring, and then boiled it. If you placed this up against a properly roasted piece of meat you would see, taste, and feel the difference.

The thing that got me was that I had been told that it saved money. How on earth did it save money? It was the same piece of meat we were using in our retail areas. Cooking food correctly does not cost any more money than cooking food incorrectly. In fact, cooking food the wrong way can actually cost more. Less yield and more waste are just a couple factors. I felt that we were just not getting it.

So the food was safe—I had to give it that. However, so was my food. We had great food-safety practices in place in the cafés; we cooked food to the proper temperature, and we cooled it as it should be done. Food safety was the most important thing we did. It was basic. All of our employees participated in a food-safety course. We monitored the cooking to ensure that no food-borne illness would occur. We served thousands of people everyday, and no one ever got sick. We did things right.

Patient Trays

I seem to you cruel and too much addicted to gluttony, when I beat my cook for sending a bad dinner. If that seems to you too trifling a cause, pray tell for what cause you would have a cook flogged?

—Marcus Valerius Martialis, Roman poet

The patient trays produced in Baltimore were sorted by specific diets and loaded onto a truck, pre-cooked and cooled. The plate comprised a main entree, a vegetable, and a starch. It was also accompanied by soup, rolls, and dessert on the tray. We would send these trays down the tray line, where they were finished with beverages, salads, and condiments. The trays were then loaded onto special retherm carts that had reheating elements built into them.

The main entree plate sat over one element, and the soup or other hot liquid was placed on the smaller element. The carts were then plugged into a receptacle and heated. The heating method was controlled by a computer system that would monitor the reheating process. It cooked the food for exactly thirty-six minutes and then held it at 140 degrees. All this was done in a huge walk-in refrigerator that kept the cold food cold while the hot food was reheating. Once the carts were unplugged, they had approximately forty-five minutes to be served. The plate itself was placed under a dome, prior to reheating, that insulated the food until it was served.

On many occasions, the food failed to heat at all. If the contact was not just right, the plate would not heat. Many times, we sent food up to the floors ice cold. Our staff was supposed to check the plate to ensure it heated, but this did not always happen. It was embarrassing when we had to go up and see the patient to try to worm our way out of a completely unacceptable situation.

These are just some of the obstacles I was faced with on my road to revolution. I had food that, even in the best situations, had major problems in its production and delivery. This poor food had been on such a long journey. It had been cooked, cooled, shipped via truck, stored, reheated by a computer, and sent upstairs a half hour later. Then the patient gets to eat it. The questions that surround this process are overwhelming. What on earth were we doing?

Now, I am sure that there are people out there who would argue this point. They would say that there is nothing wrong with cooking food this way. They would say that the food was good and that patients like it. I used to visit patients all the time when we were serving this food. Some did say it was okay, but very rarely did we hear it was great. What we did hear, repeatedly, was that the food was terrible. Our patient satisfaction scores proved it. We could not make them move upward. They sat at the bottom of all the other hospitals with which we had been compared.

Some people in the industry would say that I am being too critical, and that cook/chill is a viable means of production. I am sure in a lot of ways it is. It is used over and over again in the retail arena. Many large food companies manufacture processed foods using the cook/chill method. These items are frozen and sent off to every grocery store in America. The difference is these foods are engineered to taste good when reheated. They pack them with preservatives, salt, fat, and food additives so the average American, too busy to cook, can have a tasty meal ready for them in thirty minutes. But just take a look at the calories, grams of fat, and sodium on many of these items. This is how they are making it taste good. Who doesn't like a lot of fat and salt? Of course, it is good. The question is how good is it for your body?

Our food was not engineered. Nothing had been added to our food. It was what it was. It was a bland piece of chicken with flavorless vegetables served with parboiled white rice. The fact is that if we had cooked it properly, we could have had a good product.

Do a test for yourself. Take a piece of boneless, skinless chicken breast. Place it in an oven with nothing on it until it is cooked. Then cool it overnight. Place that same piece of chicken in your oven at 350 degrees for 36 minutes and then eat it. You be the judge. If I am wrong, let me know.

Now take another piece of chicken. Marinate it in freshly crushed garlic, a shot of fresh-squeezed lime juice, a touch of sea salt, maybe some fresh herbs, olive oil, and fresh cracked pepper. Grill it on an open flame until it is just right—juicy in the center and full of flavor. Now eat that. You will clearly see the difference. This is the point I was trying to get across to anyone who would listen—but no one was listening.

A Hospital in Virginia

Do you want to know who you are? Don't ask, act. Action will delineate and define you.

—Thomas Jefferson

By the summer of 2004, I'd had enough of the big city. I left Washington and headed south for the lovely town of Charlottesville, Virginia. I had worked in many college towns over the years, and it was good to go home. I was tired of the high-paced life and long lines of traffic that Maryland and Washington, DC had to offer. I had spent the last two years sitting on the Beltway trying to get to work, and now I was in the peaceful reigns of Monticello and Thomas Jefferson, the great vineyards that abound in Virginia, and of course, the great college bars.

The new hospital where I landed was very much like the last. It was also a cook/chill facility. We received much of our food by truck from Baltimore (this was a five-hour journey for the poor food), and the rest we cooked on premises.

The same bad practices were being implemented. I was again responsible for the retail operations, and the retail side was good—we did fantastic food. I was lucky to walk into an already well-developed retail program that was very successful in many hospitals across the country. All I had to do was make it better. The patients however were receiving the same bland food prepared by cooks who did not really know how to cook.

I remember talking to a patient one day and asking him what one thing we could do to improve the food. His reply was hire better cooks! This got me thinking on many levels.

The patients' food was dished up cold, sent to the computer retherm, and reheated. I already knew there was no way we could serve good food by this method. Something had to change. The bill of goods that someone had sold these hospitals was going to haunt them until they made some big changes. It was bad. I thought that this was the worst thing I had ever seen, It was then that I saw an article in a trade journal called "Food Service Director." I read a full-page ad about a retherm system from a big company that I used to deal with. They had a new system that could actually hold the food for three days before reheating. Even worse, they had a quote from some hospital food service director who proudly boasted she could even send up all three meals for the day at once and the computer will heat them at specific times. It would then be delivered at the appropriate time, saving labor all along the way. She boasted that her entire day's production was done by 9:00 AM.

I just about fell out of my chair. What was wrong with these people? Why would you even consider that? Who ever thought this was a good idea? I want to talk to them. Idiots like this were proud to have their food cooked three days in advance and all their meals delivered by 9:00 AM? They were a direct threat to my revolution. They just did not get it—hopefully, these folks will retire themselves out of the industry and allow people who really care about food to take over the reins.

At this hospital, we had many corporate people visiting our account. They inspected us to see if we were running the program correctly. My boss was a serious person with a passion for success. He had a strong culinary background and did try to make things better, but the problem was the cook/chill system we were using. Our patient service manager also tried to change the menu, and was able to increase our scores, but the result was the same. It was not horrible food, but it was not great food. That was the problem. We could produce okay food all day; that was easy. What was hard was producing excellent food in a hospital environment.

I remember one day we had a meeting in the kitchen, and the chef and patient services manager created a breakfast casserole made from French toast, eggs, cinnamon, and sugar. It was baked and cut into squares and then cooled. The next day it was rethermed. The result was what you would expect. Horrid!

I was excited that a movement towards good patient food had been organized, and I could not wait to see what they came up with. I looked at this horrible goop of soggy bread on the plate, hung my head, and went back to the retail area. Walking away, I mumbled to myself, "What are we doing?" It was one of the worst things I had ever seen. We were a long way from being excellent, and we were even farther from serving restaurant-quality food. They actually put that glop on the menu. I do admire that they tried. The chef was good; the manager was good; but the cooking system was bad. I did not fault them. They were at least trying.

Every day, we diligently visited patients to ask them how they liked their food. The answers were the same over and over again: the food was not good, and the patient satisfaction scores were not improving.

Meanwhile, our catering was good, and our retail operations were good. It was just our patient food that was not—the most important part of hospital food service. I kept seeing the same trend over and over. When was someone going to do something about this cook/chill nonsense? You cannot produce quality food this way. Have you ever known of a restaurant that cooks their meals a day ahead of time and then cools them? I never had. They certainly were not teaching that method in the Culinary Institute of America. I kept hearing about raising the scores, but just like all those roads that led to Rome, all those bad scores would lead to how we cooked our food.

Another Hospital in Washington

You don't need a day off. We have too much work to do. If you need me, I will be out of town on vacation. I will return your call when I get back.

—An actual voice mail message from my old boss.

In December of 2005, I was asked to go help out in one of our accounts in Washington, DC. The director of food and nutrition at this hospital had quit with very little notice, and they needed someone to take charge of the account. Someone in the hierarchy of my company thought I would be a good candidate for this position. Having spent two years in DC prior to this, I really did not want to go back. But when I got the call to go—being a good company guy—I went. I had to leave Charlottesville and go back into the madness. Truth was, I did like the city; it had a lot of history. However being up there alone was not what I wanted to do. As this was only a temporary assignment. I had to leave my wife and son behind in Charlottesville.

This hospital was a big union account with lots of problems. However, the food was *not* the cook/chill method. They served food they actually cooked in-house. My four-year long misery of looking at pre-cooked, chilled, and then rethermed food was over.

We had some decent hospital cooks. They knew nothing about cooking great food and were not too interested in excellence, but in the world of hospital food, they were not so bad. They had also been there a long time, so I knew change would be difficult for them. I would have to take things slowly—too many changes too fast would result in too many agonizing meetings with union leaders. And *I* wasn't interested in that.

I'd already spent four hours in one such meeting on the protocol of who should say good morning to whom. Apparently, a big concern of the mighty Service Employees International Union (SEIU), this was amazing to me. They claimed that anyone who came into work *behind* a co-worker was responsible for saying good morning. It was *not* the responsibility of the person who was already there (perplexing to even non-rational people). It was an extremely painful meeting to sit in, leaving me wondering what had gone wrong in America. Shouldn't everyone say good morning if they can—does this *really* need to be discussed? It was utterly ridiculous.

Given all this nonsense, I had to take it in small steps. The first thing I did was get them to batch-cook the food. This method prepares food in small quantities to ensure freshness and quality. This alone made a big difference—but it was not enough. I then began to look at *how* each meal was produced, including how the menus were put together. I could see it was a mess and would take some energy to fix.

We had a very small retail operation (it was actually a joke). I was embarrassed by what we were doing, but I could not get anyone to put money into fixing it. I was always told to wait. We had a contract issue between our company and the hospital and neither side was giving in.

We actually served food from chafing dishes. These temporary heating dishes are usually used in catering. They are heated by a canned fuel source. These are not meant to be a permanent fixture for serving food. It was unbelievable but everyone just accepted it. Keep in mind we were a global company with many excellent programs, but the food in our retail operations was pitiful. Consequently, unlike at my previous positions, most of my time here was spent on patient feeding. This was the first time in my career that I could focus full time on patient feeding; the way I saw it, it was my responsibility to serve good food. However, as the director, I was also tied up with numerous administrative tasks, negotiations with union delegates, paperwork, budgets, and costs—both labor and goods. Boring but important stuff. We had a lot of problems, especially the all-too-familiar patient satisfaction scores, which were basically in the toilet. The place was a mess; the food was awful, and the cooks were untrained.

Because of this, our corporate office sent a regional chef to help me through the holidays. We had a meeting and came up with a game plan: I would soothe the angry union employees, and he would work on the food. The employees hated the past director, who had done many things that they did not like. She was uncaring about their needs, and she stirred up animosity between management and employees. I knew that if I did not fix these problems, getting good food to the patients would be impossible. We had to raise employee morale, which was very low.

I asked the employees what had been planned for them for the Christmas holiday. This is a time when every other place I had worked had thrown a party or a nice meal for the staff. They told me nothing had been planned and that they had not even been asked about it. They had been so neglected over the last year, and they were angry about it. I decided we would put on a nice meal for them and I would buy everyone a turkey to take home. It was the least we could do.

I think they began to slightly trust me after that. I was strict, but I was also fair. They soon learned if they came to work on time, did their jobs, and treated each other and management with respect, we would all get along just fine. I also showed them that this was a two-way street, holding myself and my managers to the same standards. It was clear this had never been done before—the reaction from the staff was immediate and positive.

The corporate chef was supposed to help me train the cooks. That was his job. I had always wanted restaurant quality food in a hospital setting, and I believed with the help of this chef and the fact of a very small retail operation we could focus on just that. Instead, the chef did most of the work himself. The food was good, but he was not training anyone. The union cooks just went about their business. They looked at it as someone else doing their work, and they were just fine with that.

The chef worked with me for about two months. As his time with me came to a close, I asked him how his training had gone. He told me he was just trying to get the food out; he had no time to train. I asked him when the time came for him to leave, how the food was going to look any different when he spent no time actually training the cooks, laying out responsibilities, and setting standards. I knew I would be back to square one once he left. My cooks were going to take the easiest route possible, because they did not care about quality food. They seemed more interested in fighting management and flexing their union muscles. We had brought this chef in to train the cooks, and since he did not, he did very little to drive our program.

I wanted to change the menu again, so I met with my team. The managers were trying to do what was best. They worked hard, but they were so consumed with employee issues that they looked at a menu change as a bad Idea. They kept coming up with excuses and putting it off. I had no support from people below me or above me. I had to do this on my own. Finally, I decided to issue a mandate stating that we were going to change the menu and nothing short of a meteor hitting the US Capitol would stop us. Our scores were not moving up, and we had the same problems repeatedly.

As I was putting together the new menu, we were also starting a new type of room service. This meant sending our room service staff to the patient rooms to take their orders and verbally describe the menus to the patients. The associates would then go back to the kitchen and actually assemble the trays. The thought was that this would give the employees a feeling of ownership, causing them to remember the patients and ensure they got what they needed. We ran a pilot program on two different floors, and the results were great. The patients loved it, as well as the nursing staff. We planned to implement this system hospital-wide, but we had many union hurdles to get through first.

Once I put together my new menu, we had an all-hospital tasting one day. We invited the administration and all the nursing floors. We did chicken parmesan, grilled salmon, fresh tossed pasta with spinach, and chicken with sun-dried tomatoes. We offered items like herb-crusted pork loin with a Merlot demi-glace, chicken breast stuffed with apples and currants, fresh salads, and homemade soups. We revamped our children's menu and began to look at our heart-healthy meals. This was going to be special. This was a menu that would define us and finally bring restaurant-quality food into a hospital setting. The problem was that only the Emergency Department showed up. Not one person from the hospital leadership showed up. I could not believe it. No one cared.

I knew that day and at that moment that I needed to leave. I was surrounded by too many people who did not care about the patients or the food we were serving. The administration was not happy about the scores, but did not even have the common decency to show up and see what we were doing about it.

I plugged away for a few more months. Our patient satisfaction scores were much higher than they had been; the employees were happier; the place was cleaner. I felt I had done some good. But I was tired and wanted to go home.

The most important thing I took with me was the understanding of the absolute necessity to train our employees better. We want them to be excellent, and we want great food, but the problem was that we as a company were not training them to be excellent. Many companies have great training programs, but their execution is terrible. I lived it and I know much of it is pure rhetoric. These programs are so watered-down by the time they reach the line employee they become useless. The people who come up with these programs have the best intentions, but by the time these ideas trickle down to accounts nationwide, they are vastly different than what was first put on paper. I had a corporate chef for two months, and he never put one thing in place to make our program better for the long run. I knew I had to come up with a better plan. I needed a training program that worked. The early version of the "Black Hat Chef" was conceived. But it would still take a lot of work before I got there.

The University of North Carolina

Certain things in life are more important than the usual crap that everyone strives for.

—James Taylor

After a year in DC, a place I did not want to be, I left the company, headed south, and got away from the madness. Again.

I had spent the last nine months living in an apartment in Arlington, with my wife and stepson still in Charlottesville, Virginia. It was a hard life, commuting on weekends and being alone during the week. I had had enough. It was time to go home. But I left Washington with a heavy heart. I felt that maybe if I had stayed I could have fixed the situation; however that was not meant to be.

Angelo Mojica, my boss from my first tour of duty in Washington, had relocated to the University of North Carolina Hospitals (UNCH) and was trying to get me to move down there. It was a perfect fit. He is an extremely talented person who has a great outlook on life. I was comfortable with him, and I knew he cared about quality; he had the same vision that I did. We both wanted to serve great food.

UNCH had a brand new retail program going in place, and I was good at that. It was where I had excelled over the years, and so I was excited to build an entire retail program from the ground up. My family packed the truck and we headed back to North Carolina, the state where I had spent my army years. I liked it then, and I knew it would be a good fit for my family.

UNCH is a huge place. It has 800 beds, and being a teaching hospital, has many challenges. There are over 750 resident doctors, 8,000 employees, and scores of visitors. It is one of the largest hospitals in the state, and being right on campus at the University of North Carolina at Chapel Hill, it is an exciting place to work. I loved being there and was proud that I had been chosen to do this job. I had come a long way and been through a lot. I really felt that this was a great opportunity for me.

The first thing we did was create our own in-house brands. In the contract world, there are two types of food concepts: *national brands* (like Chick-Fil-A, Taco Bell, Quiznos, etc.) or *in-house brands*. Each food service contract company has its own in-house brand. They develop these brands in concert with the national brands. National brands have high royalty fees and commissions that are challenging to the bottom line. The lure of these brands is obvious: they have national advertisements, a loyal following, and brand recognition. It is a safe bet to bring a Chick-Fil-A into an operation, because people will come for it.

The downside is that most brands get old and tired. How many times can you eat at Quiznos? I know this first hand, as the building I lived in during my time in Arlington had a Quiznos. I ate there all the time. To this day, I can never go back to one. I was overloaded with Quiznos.

In a hospital setting, your customers are mostly employees. These folks eat there all the time. Our world of food service is unlike restaurants or hotels. We see the same people every day. This makes us even more committed to changing our menus frequently. National brands begin to suffer as customers get tired of the same old thing. House brands allow broader freedom. They are not tied down to long contracts and can be changed at will.

The in-house brands we created were progressive, offered great food, and allowed our customers to choose from a variety of options.

Bandaleros
GOURMET BURRITOS

Bandaleros

This concept came from years of working with my *compadres* in Arizona. I had spent eight years immersing myself in Latin cuisine, which is so prevalent in the Southwest. All of my cooks were from various parts of Mexico, Central and South America. I quickly learned that Mexico has a very diverse food culture. Northern states served vastly different food than the southern states. It was a whole new world opened up to me, and I was digging it.

I learned that *chilaquiles* were by far the best breakfast food I had ever had—simple, but very good. I learned how to make tamales, all types of burritos, pork *carnitas, moles, arroz con pollo, papusas, carne asada, ropa vieja, tortas,* and many more incredible foods that I had never tried before. I fell in love with Latin foods and I still consider it the best food on earth.

During this exploration of Latin foods, I came across a type of shredded beef called *machaca.* You cook top rounds of beef with chilies, tomatoes, garlic, onions, and stock. Then simmer until it shreds. It can be put into burritos or tacos, served with eggs for breakfast, or just eaten by itself. It is hot, spicy, and delicious. Beef machaca would become the cornerstone for my *Bandaleros* concept. When I was developing the brands for UNCH, Angelo wanted a Mexican burrito–style concept that rivaled Chipotles, Qdoba, or Moe's Southwestern Grill. I had spent years studying this food and I knew I could do it. Within a week, *Bandaleros* was born.

We now serve Beef Machaca, Pork Carnitas, Chipotle Marinated Chicken and Carne Asada in our concepts menu. Each is served with cilantro and lime-infused jasmine rice, black beans, pintos, and four freshly made salsas. This brand is now in two hospitals. The food is always fresh, and it is truly authentic. My cooks in Arizona would be proud of what we have done. It is the best in-house brand that I have created.

Continental Traders

Continental Traders

In every hospital, there is a "hot line." This is where foods like turkey and dressing, meatloaf, baked chicken, and lasagna are served. It is also where you find vegetables, mashed potatoes, rice, gravy, and rolls. This station is necessary in hospitals, as many customers are looking for simple, comfort food. When I developed Continental Traders, I wanted something more. My vision was that we would travel the continents and bring together a flavor that would rival any restaurant. I envisioned worlds of flavors brought together in a single concept.

The first thing was to make the staple foods, like meatloaf and roasted chicken, the best they could be. The concept of outdated cafeteria-style food had to go. Things like Jell-O, pimento cheese sandwiches, and soggy, overcooked vegetables had to go away and never come back.

We wrote the menus to make that happen. We offered grilled rib-eye steaks, blackened catfish, jambalaya, pork loin stuffed with sausage, spinach and wild rice, lamb shanks, pan-seared scallops served with a white wine butter sauce, *chimichurri* pork, beef on weck, braised ox tails, turkey mole and specialty soups like *posole* and classic French onion soup served with crusty baguettes topped with gruyere cheese.

These were not typical hospital menu items, and it excited our customers. They had never seen anything like it in a workplace. At UNCH, our retail sales doubled in a year.

We also began to work on how our vegetables and starches were prepared. We got rid of all canned vegetables and eliminated most frozen. We emphasized fresh vegetables cooked in small batches; then served them immediately. We did things like grilled eggplant with roasted garlic and olive oil. We served fresh steamed broccoli, fire-roasted asparagus, and *calabacitas* (a blend of roasted corn, squash, and onions). We were serving food that you could find in the best restaurants.

We used real mashed potatoes! I cannot even believe that I just wrote that. Many hospitals today use instant mashed potatoes—just add water.

This was not the path we were going down. We actually serve two types of mashed potatoes—fresh, redskin mashed potatoes and roasted garlic mashed potatoes. We used rice varieties like jasmine, arborio, and basmati. These are far superior to the "converted" white rice that you see in most hospitals.

Our food was better, and it was beginning to gain real traction with our customers.

Cosimos

Cosimos was a straightforward program. We were going to offer fresh made pizza, stromboli, calzone, and other specialty Italian dishes. I wanted it to be authentic. I had cooked many years in Italian restaurants, and I knew the basics. I understood that a marinara sauce must be fresh and flavorful. Pasta had to be al dente. We used the freshest herbs and imported cheeses. I wanted this to be special. I wanted a true taste of Italy.

Typical hospitals offer pizza served with very little variety. They often just do a vegetarian, plain cheese, and pepperoni or sausage pizzas. We offer pizzas like Philly steak and cheese, pancetta and arugula, barbecued chicken pizza with red onion and cilantro, pesto chicken, white pizza, and Cancún grilled shrimp pizza.

Our specialty entrees include items such as chicken marsala, shrimp scampi, tortellini with Parma ham, artichokes, and Italian sausage. I frequently do a classic pork-and-peppers-over-linguine; or beef *braciole*, a stuffed roulade of beef, so delicious that it warms the soul. We cook our pasta fresh daily and only add the freshest ingredients available. Items such as spaghetti and meatballs, sausage and peppers, grilled chicken with penne pasta in an Alfredo sauce, shrimp fra diavlo, and pasta pomodora are just a few of the classic pasta dishes we serve daily.

Of course, Caesar salads, pasta fagioli, and rosemary focaccia bread are available to round off the meal. Cosimos is certainly different from what you would expect in a hospital.

Mezza Luna

This was our masterpiece brand. A group of us traveled to New York City to check out the food scene. We boarded a plane at Raleigh-Durham International Airport and left for JFK. When we got to New York, we were on a mission. We ate at as many different restaurants, bistros, pizza joints, street vendors, and beer halls as we could. We ended up at Les Halles in Manhattan. Anthony Bourdain is the "at-large" chef there, and he is actually the inspiration for this book. Our journey in Manhattan was a culinary dream come true.

During our visit to New York, we took a train to the Culinary Institute of America in Hyde Park to visit their new café called the Apple Pie Bakery café. We brought one of our cooks on this trip. He was interested in going to school there, so we thought it would be a good opportunity for him to see the school first hand. On the way back we had an hour to kill at the train station, so Angelo had a great idea: he went and got some beer to help kill the time.

When we got on the train, we busted out the beer and started to plan our new food concept. We did not have a name yet but we knew what we wanted. While we were drinking the beers, I had this bad feeling that what we were doing was not legal. At one stop, New York's finest boarded the train. They looked at us, and I said, "That's it; they're going to arrest us," but all they said was have a cold one on us, and they walked away. Angelo was born and raised in NYC and he knew much more about the way things worked than I did. In New Hampshire, we would have been put in jail for drinking in public. God bless NY; they see things differently.

I had not been in Manhattan in years and had forgotten just how good the food was. It was truly inspiring. We ate great food, drank good beer, and then ate more food. I was loving it.

What we learned from our trip was that the City had a huge market for fresh-made salads. They were everywhere we went. They were topped with hundreds of ingredients. We saw items like octopus, duck breast, grilled chicken, tenderloin, flank steak, shrimp, salmon, artichokes, and calamari. The toppings never seemed to end. We knew after only a short time in Manhattan that we needed to do this. It was a healthy option that our customers would love. We knew that if New York, New York, was doing it, it was a trend that we should take a serious look at. And it would work perfectly in a hospital setting.

We packed up our notes and left for North Carolina. We felt confident that we had a good program. One year later we opened Mezza Luna at both UNCH and Rex Hospital in Raleigh. At the time of our trip to New York, a contractor was managing Rex's food and nutrition department. Even though Rex is part of the UNC system it was not on our radar. We had no idea when developing this brand that just one year later our food empire would grow to include another 440 bed hospital.

It was great to see Mezza Luna actually happening. This new café was basically created while traveling on a train from Poughkeepsie to NYC over a twelve-pack of Sam Adams beer and writing down ideas on a note pad. To see this idea come to fruition a year later was very satisfying to me.

The folks at UNCH and Rex really made this work and the results were great. We wanted a gas-fired pizza oven serving signature pizza, calzones, and flatbreads. We wanted homemade soups, paninis, and a fresh bakery concept. We wanted New York–style bagels with many spreads to choose from, and we wanted awesome fresh-tossed salads made to order. We had made it work, and it rivaled anything in any hospital or upscale food court anywhere. It actually puts many restaurants to shame. It is that good.

Mezza Luna now offers over fifty toppings with your choice of salad greens. We offer over ten dressings and fresh-baked rolls.

Our house brands repertoire also includes a smoothie concept named Max Mangoes and display cooking called Chefs-in-Motion. All these brands are unique to UNCH and Rex Hospital. Our brands rival any other company's brands in quality of food and variety. We are proud of them and our customers keep coming back for more.

Patient Feeding at the UNC Hospitals

I will use Jedi mind tricks on them. They will think that these are the droids they are looking for.

—Angelo Mojica, Director Food and Nutrition, UNC Hospitals, when asked how we were going to get this new menu past the dietitians

After a year and a half of operations in our retail venues, it was time to move on. I felt that I had done what I could to drive sales and create great food for our customers. I had my old friend Ryan Miller running the operation now, and my time had come. Ryan had been my partner in crime for many years. The stories we could tell about our journeys together most people would never believe. We worked together in Arizona, Alabama, Virginia, and now North Carolina, all within a span of ten years. I knew my retail operation was in good hands, as Ryan is one of those guys who sees the vision and gets it done. At first, I was very protective over my retail operations. It was hard to let go. Ryan and I would often get mad at each other during the day, but as usual, we would belly up at some bar later and forget all the bad feelings that had occurred during the day. We had seen too much over the years to let bullshit get in the way of our friendship.

But I was ready to move onto another project; I wanted a more important puzzle to solve. I wanted to make a big difference in people's lives. What I really wanted to do was concentrate on patient food. I wanted to finish what I had started in Washington. I knew that I could make permanent changes in the way patients were being fed.

Patient food at UNCH was not bad. Angelo was very motivated to make things better. He had done some of the groundwork in fixing the food, but being the director of a large department, he could not focus full time like I could.

The first thing I looked at was how patients on general nutrition therapy (a regular diet) were being fed. I had discovered over the years that the cooks would prepare one version of the meal that would cover all of the diet spreads. This meal could be served to the vast majority of patients.

The diets in a hospital are prescribed by the physician. You may be put on a heart-healthy diet, a renal diet, low sodium, two-gram sodium, *neutropenic*[5], pureed, chopped, or diabetic. There are additional types of diets, but most would fall into these categories.

Each diet has some restriction that we must follow. Heart-healthy diets must be just that: they must fall in line with the American Heart Association's guidelines. Our diabetic diet must have a certain amount of carbohydrates per day, and our renal diets must be able to support people with kidney failure. The guidelines were strict, and we had to abide.

What I learned about these diets was that when a patient came in to the hospital, most knew nothing of restricted diets and why they were on them. Our job, along with the dietitians, was to educate them. Many of them just could not accept that they were being placed on a restriction. They wanted to eat whatever they wanted. This caused a lot of problems for us, as we just could not let them do that.

Then you have the type of patients who know how to work the system and use it as a crutch. One day, I received a phone call from hospital security stating there was patient who had claimed we tried to kill her, and she wanted to speak with the director. I went to the room and found the patient surrounded by hospital staff. There was administration, patient relations, nurses, doctors, and security. This patient stated that she was a diabetic and we had served her apple juice. She claimed that if she had drunk it, she could have died. "Don't you know I am a diabetic?" she cried repeatedly. It was an incredible scene.

Ridiculous is a word I use often, but this scenario was more than I could handle. I was actually at a loss for words, which by the way, is rare for me. This woman was over six hundred pounds. Her body was so big, I did not know where the bed ended and she began. I almost began to laugh. Here she was claiming that a four-ounce juice was going to kill her.

5 Neutropenic diets are served to people with weakened immune system. This requires that all food is cooked thoroughly to protect them from harmful bacteria.

It took every bit of energy for me not to say, "Hey lady, what about the six hundred pounds? Maybe that's the problem. Lose some weight and don't worry about the juice. Did you ever think that maybe you are a diabetic because you weigh so much?"

Four ounces of juice to her would have been like an M1 Abrams tank running over a garden hose. It would have never even been noticed. Instead, I apologized and told her that we would take extra caution on her future meals. She continued to play it up and probably got a free hospital stay out of it.

Unfortunately, we deal with people who grossly overreact or try to get something for nothing—they have learned how to work the system and they do it well. For the most part, however, our patients are just trying to get better so that they can go home.

Patient diets were now part of my world—that's what I asked for—and I would have to deal with their needs. I accepted this and wanted to figure out how to make each diet the best that I could. They all deserved good food, and that was what I was being paid to do.

If you look at the entire hospital population, most are on regular diets. This means they can eat just about anything. They have no sodium or fat restrictions. However, if you only served one "version" of a meal, the regular diets would end up eating what the cardiac, low-sodium, and low-fat people were eating.

This meant that when we cooked turkey, mashed potatoes, gravy, and a vegetable, they were all low sodium and low fat. It was not what a "healthy" patient would want to eat. In fact, it was exactly where the stereotypes of hospital food came from. I asked the patient service manager to have lunch with me. We were going to eat exactly what a patient eats. We got our trays and sat down to eat. I wanted to be the patient and experience for myself what they were eating.

I started with a low-sodium chicken noodle soup. It had been made from scratch and did have good possibilities, but it tasted very bland. It had absolutely no flavor. I then had the turkey, mashed potatoes, gravy, and broccoli. The turkey had not been roasted properly. It was pale and overcooked, very dried out. The potatoes were instant and had absolutely no flavor. It was like eating Styrofoam or some kind of plumber's putty. The gravy was made from instant powder—you know, the kind you just add water to—and it also had no salt. The broccoli was ridiculously over-cooked and it was "broccoli cuts," a frozen tear-jerking form of broccoli that is mostly stems. The only thing good was the roll, which of course was served with a no-fat margarine spread.

The meal was a disaster. Given that over half of our patient population had no dietary restrictions, why were we serving this *restricted* type of food? The answer was simple: The cooks are too lazy to cook food appropriate for the diets, and most management teams see two types of the same food as a cost—they do not want to spend the money.

Those same management teams are also the ones that are constantly scurrying around visiting patients, trying to get their scores up. They do not see what the root problem is—it is the food. It's quite simple: if you want your patients to think your food is excellent, then serve excellent food. If you live in a world of denial and try to get patients to think your food is good by talking to them and trying to convince them, well that is like putting lipstick on a pig. It just does not make the food better.

My first obstacle was the registered dietitians (RDs) because they look at food differently than a chef does. They see it in a clinical sense. The idea of cooking without a recipe that is calculated down to the last gram of salt is unknown to them. Food is an absolute, and every ingredient must be accounted for and analyzed. Well, this just bores me to death. I asked one of the dietitians how confident she was about the two-gram sodium diets. "Are they needed and do they really matter?" Her response was that patients with a certain type of medical problem that need a limited amount of sodium must be put on this. It aids in their recovery. Now, I am sure it does.

There are people smarter than me that go to school for ten years to become docs. They certainly know better than I do on this subject but I do know that too much sodium is not good for you. My argument was, and still is, when is the last time you saw a gram scale in a major production kitchen? Do you really think that there are exactly two grams of sodium in that patient's meal? I have the answer … No!

I have spent thousands of hours cooking side by side with hospital cooks, and I know getting them to follow specific recipes can be a huge undertaking. To get them to ensure that exactly two grams of sodium are on that patient's tray is impossible. It just does not happen like that. Most hospitals, just to be on the safe side, remove salt from their recipes entirely.

Being the good manager that I am, I did have to follow some guidelines in my menu development. There are viable medical reasons that patients should not be fed anything they want. Diabetic patients must control their carbohydrates and eat at specific times. I certainly would not send southern fried chicken to a cardiac floor. Nor would I send bananas or tomatoes to a patient with kidney failure. There are rules that we needed to follow.

However, I did want to stretch the limits as far as I could. Being a chef, I wanted as much flavor in the food as I could possibly have, but I knew that added salt and fat were not going to get me anywhere. The dietitians outnumbered me, and I knew from experience not to make them mad. They are like bees—if you rattle the hive, you will get stung. I knew I could not win that battle. So, I decided on another course of action.

Luckily, for me, our chief clinical dietitian understood about good food. She was not a chef, but wanted to see results in the patient scores. She allowed me to create recipes that she could review. Our offices were right next to each other, and when I got a recipe done, I would take it over to her. Our recipe software would show the number of calories, sodium, potassium, fat, etc. She would hand it back and say, "Too much salt," or "Too many carbohydrates," etc. I would go sulking back to my office to give it another try.

As a chef, I knew that good food did not have to be laden with salt or fat. I had learned this fact years ago at the Culinary Institute of America. I began to look at our heart-healthy menu in a different light. What if I used things like marinades, fresh herbs, roasted garlic, and fresh citrus juices to get the flavor profiles I was looking for? I would show those RDs that the world of chefs and the dietitians can coexist.

I rewrote the whole menu with an entire "heart-healthy" section. It was bold; it was different, and I think I had finally found a way to get restaurant-quality food past the "sodium police" and make our patients happy.

Our Heart-Healthy Menu includes items such as these:

Beef en Brochette

Beef tenderloin, marinated in fresh squeezed limejuice, rosemary, garlic, olive oil, cracked black pepper, and a touch of sea salt. Skewered with green peppers, mushrooms, tomatoes, and red onions.

Ginger Marinated Salmon

Fresh salmon fillets grilled with fresh ginger, lime zest, and cilantro.

Calypso Chicken

Chicken breast marinated with fresh pineapple, mangoes, cilantro, and jalapeño. Served with a roasted tomato confit. Topped with Down-Island salsa.

Pretzel-Crusted Pork Tenderloin

Pork tenderloin rolled in crushed sourdough pretzels and pan-seared. Served with a red wine, whole-grain mustard, and roasted shallot demi-glace.

Blue Ridge Chicken

Marinated and grilled chicken breast topped with charred baby spinach, a slice of fresh mozzarella cheese, diced tomatoes, garlic, and fresh basil. Served with a red bell pepper coulis.

Chili-Rubbed Chicken Fajitas

Ancho and guajillo chilies–rubbed chicken breast grilled and served with black beans, jasmine rice, and fresh *pico de gallo*. Served with warmed flour tortillas.

Grilled BBQ Pork Loin

Grilled pork loin mopped with our house-made peach and chipotle barbecue sauce.

Asian Lettuce Wraps

Grilled chicken, Thai chilies, garlic, bamboo shoots, and water chestnuts simmered in a spicy broth. Served with crisp lettuce leaves and a dipping sauce. Accompanied with a crisp cucumber and carrot salad.

Mediterranean Tilapia en Papillotte

Tilapia filet, grape tomatoes, fresh oregano, snipped green beans, olives, lemon juice, and julienned zucchini, wrapped in paper and baked to seal in the natural juices and flavors. Served with a toasted almond brown rice pilaf.

These were not typical menu items that you would see on a patient menu. We were proud of these, and our patients loved the new direction we were heading.

The beauty was that since I had a low-fat, low-sodium menu, I could also allow the regular-diet patients to eat food that rivaled any restaurant in town. We now had menus that could satisfy not only the dietitians, but most importantly, the patients themselves.

We offered chicken marsala, Asian beef and broccoli stir-fry, sautéed chicken breast with lemon and fresh thyme, home-style pot roast, and stuffed pork loin to our regular patients. They loved it, and our patient satisfaction scores began to move up.

I also looked hard at the breakfast meal. I learned over the years that many patients have a busy day of testing, rehab, MRI scans, and other things that can prevent them from eating on a normal schedule. Patients are often put on NPO temporarily—meaning they cannot eat or drink anything for some period of time while testing is underway. When patients get off NPO, they are very hungry. Often, the first meal they can get is breakfast.

Our breakfast menu had plenty of room for improvement. We served basics like scrambled eggs—something I had cringed over for many years. We served pancakes and French toast, but not on the same day. We served grits, oatmeal, farina, bacon, sausage, and grilled ham. That was about it.

A New Breakfast Menu

I wanted to do more. I wanted a true, restaurant experience with our breakfast meal. I wanted what any good breakfast joint would serve. Why did we have to serve such basic things? I put on huevos rancheros, a classic Mexican-food dish with eggs, cheddar cheese, and refried beans topped with our fresh-made pico de gallo and chopped cilantro, served in a fried corn tortilla bowl. We also offered breakfast parfaits made with fresh blueberries, vanilla yogurt, and house-made granola.

I developed a breakfast skillet that had potatoes, bacon, eggs, and cheese all served in a casserole dish. I added banana-nut, buckwheat, and blueberry pancakes to the menu. We serve a breakfast Monte Cristo, which is a sandwich made with honey ham and Swiss cheese, dipped into French toast batter, and grilled. It is then served with an orange marmalade.

We reinvented the omelet. We have over ten fillings that the patient can choose from. We serve scrambled eggs with feta cheese and tomatoes. We offer biscuits and gravy and a New York–style roll, with egg, bacon, and cheese.

I then went a step further and created our Heart-Healthy Breakfast menu. Breakfast is so typically full of fat—lots of bacon, sausage etc. I wanted our heart-healthy patients to be able to eat something other than oatmeal. I came up with a low-fat spinach, mushroom, and tomato frittata.

I added a grilled peach-and-yogurt dish that has grilled peaches splashed with balsamic vinegar, fresh-made granola, and low-fat yogurt. I created the "Breakfast Skinny," which is an open-faced breakfast sandwich with a whole-wheat English muffin, shaved low-sodium ham, egg whites, and low-fat jack cheese. It is one of our most popular menu items to date.

I even do a stuffed portabella mushroom filled with scrambled egg whites, spinach, and feta cheese. These menus are innovative, and our patients love the options they can choose from

Our breakfast menu rivals any other in town—hospital or restaurant. Our patients cannot believe that they can get these choices in a hospital setting. This was exactly what I was looking for.

I had known my entire career that this needed to be done. It was only through persistence and selling my story to anyone who would listen that things began to change. It was a long and painful journey, but it was beginning to pay off.

Things That Just Should Not Be Allowed

Forgive them Lord, they know not what they do—or that they don't care. Has to be one or the other.

—Okay, I took a few liberties here.
Probably get struck by lightning ... Sorry, God!

Over the years, I have seen some incredible things take place in hospital kitchens. I could write a separate book just on that subject alone. I have seen perfectly good food destroyed by cooks who a year ago—or a week ago—used to be the dishwashers. I have seen burnt, undercooked, flavorless food being served without any remorse. It's as if the standards were set to do just the very minimal and nothing more. I wanted to change this mentality, and in order to do this, I had to outlaw a few things.

Fruit Cocktail

What in the world is this? I have never seen anything more insulting. I've never liked fruit cocktail, even when I was a kid. The grapes are macerated, the peaches are mushy, the maraschino cherries are awful, and what in the world is that square white thing? This had to go.

I now serve a fresh fruit cup with ... wait for it ... fresh fruit! We serve cantaloupe, honeydew, pineapple (when allowed by diet restrictions), fresh strawberries, and blueberries. We garnish it with fresh mint and, if the patient so requests, we shave Belgian chocolate over it. It is fresh and inviting. Canned fruit cocktail is not my version of a fruit cup. I do however have to keep it on my menu for those patients too sick to eat fresh fruit. I do not allow it be served to anyone who does not meet that criterion. Neither should you!

Dried Parsley

This is also just plain ridiculous. Who thought of this? Fresh-chopped parsley has a wonderful aroma and taste and is available all year long in most places. It is used in many of our dishes. I have told my cooks that dried parsley should never be used—it is horrible and just should not exist—period. In fact, whenever I go into someone else's kitchen and I see it, I secretly throw it out. The worst thing is that chefs who read this book who work outside of a hospital setting may never have known that there is such a thing as dried parsley. Sadly, there is.

Pimento Cheese

Sorry to all you Southerners, but I just don't get it!

Canned or Bottled Salsa

We can do better! Our *Bandaleros* concept makes four fresh salsas a day. Use one of them.

Jell-O

Tried to fight this one, but too many patients need it, as many can only eat liquids. If you are serving this to *any* other patient, you need to stop—my god, it's Jell-O! It is not anything you would ever see in a restaurant. If you eat Jell-O in a restaurant, you need to venture out more, find a better place.

Toast

We do serve it—but toast can never be good in hospital settings. It is always soft and rubbery by the time it gets to the patient. The *only* way we could do good toast would be to put a toaster in the room—probably not a good idea

Oven "Grilled" Chicken

This is when the cooks place frozen chicken on a sheet pan and then throw it in the oven. It emerges as a lifeless, overcooked piece of rubber. Everywhere I have been I have seen this sinful act. It is just plain wrong. Our cooks now marinate our chicken and *grill* them, as they should. The funny thing about grilled chicken is that somewhere along the line it has to be grilled. I have never seen anything grilled in an oven. It just does not work. Stop doing it.

Dried Basil

Dried basil cannot be substituted for fresh basil. Not on anything. Can you imagine a caprese salad with dried basil? This is not going to work. Buy fresh basil and do everyone a favor.

Canned Vegetables.

Just stop! They are not good for anything. Cannot even think of one reason why I would ever use them.

Frozen Broccoli Cuts

These should only be served in prisons. They are mostly stems and are not good for anyone ... well, except prisoners. Try fresh steamed broccoli florets instead.

Dried Rosemary

If you like sharp needles jabbing through the roof of your mouth use dried rosemary. If you are looking for that wonderful flavor that rosemary can bring to your food, then use fresh rosemary. Grow your own herb garden or buy it from your produce supplier. It is cheap and plentiful. The difference in flavor is unbelievable.

The Multi-Purpose Knife

These are knives that look like what you would get when you open a bank account. They are serrated, curved like a scimitar, and many hospital cooks use them for everything. They are very cheaply made and are always dull.

The cooks, especially ones who have been there for many years, will look at a chef's knife and say, "I am not using that big ol' knife." It kills me to hear this. They do not use cutting boards but hold a cucumber in their hands and cut slice by slice with these horrible knives—very slowly. It is painful to watch them use these knives. I have outlawed them and not one of my cooks uses these ridiculous things.

I have invested so much money over the years providing proper knives to my cooks it is not even funny. There is a different knife for every different job. You cannot dice an onion with a paring knife. We constantly train our cooks on the proper use of knives so that they know how to use them to do the job. However, it was very difficult to change them.

Look around your kitchens. Do multi-purpose knives exist? If they do, you need to invest some time training your cooks on proper knife skills.

The "Boiled Hamburger" and Its Evil Twin Sister, the "Boiled Chicken"

These foods just absolutely kill me. They are the worst things that occur in our retail operations. But they happen everywhere I have ever been, with the exception of UNCH. The grill cooks will cook up twenty to thirty burgers and chicken breasts ahead of time. Then they submerge them in a pan with a little beef base (or chicken base) and water. Then they place the pan on the grill. The water begins to boil and the meat begins to die a very rapid death.

The reality of this horrible method is lazy cooking by cooks who don't care enough to serve a good product. The excuse they use is that the customers will not wait for a burger to cook from the raw state. When they get an order for the burger, they pull one out of its greasy deathtrap and place it on the grill. Then they add cheese and, wham, within thirty seconds, you have a greasy, overcooked, and soggy burger. Horrible.

My solution is to have the burger meat thawed, so that you are not throwing a frozen, rock-hard hockey puck on the grill, better yet, hand form your burgers from fresh ground beef. Tell the customers that you are cooking their burgers fresh, and it should only be a few minutes. Better yet, you know when your rush is; place a few burgers on the grill, and get them started. You will sell them all.

There is no burger place in the world that boils its burgers. McDonalds serves millions a day; theirs are never boiled. They just know how to do it.

Please. If this is happening in your hospital, make it your main mission in life to stop it. It is bad and it is lazy and there is no reason that your cooks should be doing this. It is utter nonsense.

These are just a few of the things I have outlawed. In order to make changes in hospital food, we must stop thinking of *the way it has always been done*. We are in the business of feeding people. We need to do it with restaurant-quality food in mind. Be the change!

Black Hat Chefs

Hey, soldier, keep running; don't walk—
airborne shuffle if you have to.

—A Black Hat Instructor in my face on a ten-mile run
Bravo Company, US Army Parachute Infantry School,
Fort Benning, GA, 1986

The airborne shuffle was most certainly not a dance. And here I was—hopping to it again.

The situation I had gotten myself into now was serving food that rivaled any restaurant in town. The problem was that I did not have the quality of cooks that restaurants have to keep it going.

Restaurants and hotels lure aspiring culinarians. Hospitals are the last place an aspiring chef wants to work. If someone had asked me upon graduating from the Culinary Institute where I wanted to work, a hospital would have been the last place I would have ever thought of. Hospital cooks just think of it as a job. It was hard to get them to understand what we were trying to do with food and cooking, but hiring chefs at salaries outside our pay range was not going to happen.

Given this, I knew I had to come up with a plan to sustain the hard work I had already done. Then I remembered the culinary training idea that I wanted to develop during my second tour in DC. I realized that serious training would break the culture of the health care cooks. These cooks needed training more than anyone I had ever met in the industry. The time was about to come.

The name *Black Hat Chef* came from my days at Fort Benning Airborne Infantry School. Fort Benning was where the army's jump school was located—where they taught soldiers how to parachute from airplanes. I had been a scared nineteen-year old, thrust into a world that I could never have imagined. We jumped from mock airplanes, thirty-foot towers, and finally, a C-141 aircraft.

The instructors who taught the school wore black baseball caps with their rank and the wings of an airborne soldier on their hat. They were called the Black Hats. These guys were unstoppable. They were the most hard-core, totally driven people I had ever met—before or since.

The Black Hats could run all day and they did. They ran *us*. We would run eight–ten miles a day in full gear. We did pushups until our arms became rubber and we could physically not go on. We were constantly being harassed. It never stopped. Even when we got back to the barracks, it was just another opportunity for them to mess with us. But it made us strong, and it taught me if you wanted to be the best, you had to earn it.

We went from a battalion of 500 soldiers to just over 300 when we graduated. Most had quit in disgrace. These Black Hats were tough. They had the daily "quitters" line up in our evening formation so that we all could see them. The Special Forces in the military, including the Airborne, are all volunteers. They certainly allow you to drop out if you cannot handle the training. The last thing the army wants is for someone to freeze in the door of an aircraft that is deploying combat Airborne soldiers. People die when that happens. They would rather you not be there. Quitting the Airborne does not mean that you get out of the service; it just means that you could not handle special training, and you will be sent back to the line units *as a failure.*

I had hated what I'd gotten myself into, but there was no way in hell I was going to be one of those guys, one of those failures. I could never ever put myself into that group. I would do what I had set out to do, and that was to graduate from jump school and become a US Army Paratrooper.

Those Black Hats made a life-long impression on me. I wanted to *be* them. I wanted to be as hard charging as they were. They truly motivated me.

While I was trying to develop the culinary program at UNCH and searching for name, I noticed what our cooks were wearing. Paradoxically, they all wore black baseball caps as part of their uniform. It gave me an idea. One day, I tried it on an employee of mine, who was also an ex-paratrooper: "What about the *Black Hat Chefs*?" He knew exactly where

I was going. He too had been to that school. The Black Hats meant something special; it meant they were dedicated. It meant they were well trained. We would be the Black Hat Chefs at UNCH. The idea had a name; now I needed the program.

Years ago, while I was working with one of the big food contractors, I was selected to become a culinary trainer. I went back to my alma mater and did a whole week of Train the Trainer. The CIA was developing a culinary training program that would actually reach down to the frontline cooks. These were the people who needed it the most. We did our training, received our training materials, and went out into the workplace. I was the campus executive chef at Auburn University in Alabama at the time as well as the area's training chef. I was so excited about this program; I could not wait to begin it.

My first training session was met with resistance. The "non-food people" of the company saw it as a waste of time. The training sessions were quick and had little impact on overall performance. The cooks looked at it with disdain and management would not go along with it. I tried to get this program launched at four other universities, and each time, it met the same fate.

I remember that one of our tasks was to track our food cost and report back to the corporate office on how this program affected overall cost. I kept track of our progress for six months, and I reported back to them with my data. They told me that of all the twenty-five or so culinary trainers they had out in the field, I was the only one who had done what was asked. It was amazing. I began to see then that people said they cared about good food, but they really did not want to do the work. Producing good food takes a lot of work. It was not going to come easy.

My *Black Hat Chef* program was going to be different. I did not have the vast resources of a large company to get this going. I could not send my cooks for a weeklong training to the CIA, and I could not spend an untold amount of money on training materials. Again, I was on my own. What I did have was a huge passion for food and an understanding of where I wanted to go. That would have to be enough.

I developed the first draft of the *Black Hat Chef Program* with the help of my co-worker and fellow chef, Betsy Thomas. She kept me on track and made it realistic. She also corrected the misspellings and horrible formatting that I usually do with Word documents. Without her, the Black Hat Chef program would not have been as successful as it is today.

My idea was to have a four-tiered program that would focus on culinary foundations, the very essence of what makes someone a good cook. It was designed to teach how food, when properly prepared, can be something of which to be proud. It is what we do for a living—we should be the best.

At the CIA, we went through six weeks of skills development. These classes were designed to teach students the fundamentals of cooking. We learned knife skills, how to make stocks, how to sauté, roast, poach, and boil. I would have to simplify their program for our cooks, but my plan was to put these basic skills into my training syllabus and build a program that could help us in our mission to serve great food. Knowing the basics enables a cook to build on that and do bigger and better things. Not knowing the basics leads to shortcuts and poor quality food. Poor quality food is what I had been seeing for years.

The first tier taught basic principles such as knife skills, how to *cost* a recipe, how to sauté properly, how to roast, how to make stocks, and most importantly, how to bring it all together.

At first, the cooks were hesitant to do this training. Many had been there for years and either had no motivation to learn more or they thought they knew it all already. So we made the Black Hat Chef training mandatory for all of our cooks. We were going in the direction of first-class food being served in a hospital, and they had a choice—get on the bus or get off.

In the early days of this program, we tried many different approaches on how we were going to get the cooks through the course. At first, we did two-hour training periods. That seemed to go well, but we had over thirty cooks; it was going to take forever. We met every Friday and discussed the training and how it was progressing. With the classes starting and stopping, the cooks were forgetting what we had taught them. We knew that the only way to do this was to send them to school, so to speak.

We started taking two at a time off the schedule to go for an entire week of training. They would be paid but not have any responsibilities other than the Black Hat Chef program. The cooks loved this idea—it offered a big break from their day–to-day routines. It was also invaluable to keep the path of learning continuous. The cooks were immersed in the training, and they took it seriously.

There was no one out there who devoted as many resources to training their staff as we did. It was revolutionary, and I am still proud to be part of it. I had watched this program grow from a simple idea; to see it in motion was a career landmark for me.

My first class had two cooks. We spent the week making veal stock, chicken stock, and demi-glace. They learned how to properly use their knives. They learned many of the classical cuts: battonet, julienne, dice, chiffonade, etc. All of this was so new to them. They were excited and spellbound at the many new ingredients to which they were exposed. Health-care kitchens never had items such as veal bones, radicchio, Belgian endive, goat cheese, cheesecloth, or fresh herbs. The cooks certainly never used words like *fond* (the wonderful drippings and pan remnants left by roasting or sautéing foods). They never talked about *mise-en-place* (assembling your ingredients and tools) or using terms like dry-heat cooking vs. moist-heat cooking. It was an alien world to them, and they were beginning to understand where we were coming from.

We roasted whole chickens and made pan gravy from the drippings in the pan. Our cooks were used to using powdered gravy, and they had never tasted anything like what we made. It was wonderful, full of flavor, and it was something that they had made! By midweek, they were really getting into it.

We taught them how to sauté properly. They learned that sautéed vegetables could not come from using a steamer. This was where they had done most of their cooking. They learned that high heat, low fat, and small-portion-sized pieces made up the basics of sauté. They learned how to make sauces from the fond in the sauté pan. It was so good to see them in action.

We costed out recipes and showed them how to do culinary math. This was our biggest challenge, as most of our cooks had never done anything like this before. They were amazed at how much food really cost. They had never been exposed to the financial side of food production. When they learned how much we spent on food purchases, their outlook changed. It is amazing to me how many directors keep the financial information secret from their staff.

I have always shared this information, as I feel that we are all in this together, and information, good or bad, must be shared. When we are doing well financially, I feel it is important for our staff to be part of that. It is also important to explain that financial success does not mean that everyone gets a raise (which is usually the first response I get). We have budgets to meet and equipment to buy.

Another point is that we have good months and bad months. We have to have a nest egg to fall back on when sales are low or when some piece of equipment fails or when we are asked to give free food in one of the many requests we get throughout the year. After a year of department meetings, my staff was beginning to understand how expensive it is to run a large department in a hospital. It is not cheap, and many resources go into its success.

In essence, they learned how the money came in and out of a restaurant. They were amazed at how much money was spent in a week on food. I wanted the cooks to learn that a case of tomatoes was not just a case of tomatoes—it was $38.00. (This, of course, varies by the season.) Seeing how we used hundreds of cases of tomatoes in a year, that money added up big-time. It was real dollars.

They were also amazed at how much it cost in payroll. They learned that their hourly wage was not just what the hospital paid them. There are FICA taxes that are matched per employee, unemployment insurance, and all the other benefits that came along with their pay, including in medical, vision, and dental insurance. We also offer a 403B retirement plan. All of this costs huge sums of money, much of which is unknown to the average employee. I know firsthand that there are many restaurants out there that do not offer any benefits for their employees. We pay an average of 28% above what they receive in pay. In other words, a $10.00-an-hour employee's actual cost is $12.80 per hour. Sharing this information helps employees know just what they are receiving from their employer.

The week ended with a grand dinner being served. They had to make a dish that contained menu items from the competencies we taught them. They made Chicken Breast Fine Herbes, which is a classical dish using sautéed chicken breast with chervil, tarragon, and parsley. It was served with a demi-glace that they made from the product of their veal stock classes. It was finished with cream and butter. They served it with a locally grown vegetables and a creamy risotto.

The meal was then served to the vice president of the hospital and a few other VIPs. The cooks came into the room and announced their meal. I was so proud of them. They were confident in what they were saying, and they were proud of what they had accomplished. It was a great meal, far from what they had previously been cooking. My *Black Hat Chef* program was under way and the results looked and tasted great!

Upon graduation, the cooks received their very own Black Hat Chef jacket with their name embroidered on it. They were given their own personal knives and a five hundred dollar bonus for completing the class. This was how serious we were about this. We wanted a complete buy-in, and we got it.

In honor of the Black Hats at Ft. Benning, the chefs also have one black star embroidered onto their collars. This is to signify that they had attained Black Hat Level One. It signifies their rank.

At the writing of this book, we have every cook at UNC hospitals at Black Hat Level One and are currently training them through Black Hat Level 2. In the coming months, we will begin Black Hat training throughout the system. Our goal is to have every cook go through the training. We have already seen a positive impact on how our food is prepared.

The Other Half of the Journey

The best day of your life is the one on which you decide your life is your own. No apologies or excuses. No one to lean on, rely on, or blame. The gift is yours—it is an amazing journey—and you alone are responsible for the quality of it. This is the day your life really begins.

—Bob Moawad, teacher, author, speaker and coach

So the food was cooked. It was better than it had ever been. Our cooks were walking around proud of themselves. It was working. Our patient satisfaction scores were going up and our retail sales were blowing away anything we had ever predicted. The patients scores had indeed moved up, but they had not moved up enough. It was still not where we wanted it. It was not good enough.

Cooking the food was just half of our battle. In a hospital setting, there are many obstacles between the patient and the food they are about to eat. The other half of the journey is, in many ways, harder then actually cooking the food.

We have to get each meal to the patient before it gets cold. In a hotel room-service operation, you have as few as eight–ten trays at a time going up; however we have up to thirty trays being sent at once. This takes a lot of time to serve. If we could just throw the tray in there like a paperboy throwing a newspaper, we could get it done quickly, but of course, we can't do that. Our servers have to spend some time with each patient. Some want their bed table adjusted, or they want to have the meal explained.

They may have a comment or a complaint or just want to talk. Our staff is trained to attend to their needs, and sometimes it takes longer than it should. If this happens with all thirty patients, it could be an hour before that employee gets back downstairs for another cart. If it takes too long, the food begins to suffer.

I have broken down some of the biggest challenges we face every day. Our goal as managers is to minimize the distractions that occur and try to make tray delivery more efficient. It is (to say the least) very painful at times.

The sense of urgency that most of our employees lack is what makes providing good service harder than it has to be. There are some employees who will do everything they can to get to the floors as soon as possible, but there are some who tend to take their time. This behavior is what we needed to stop. This is their job, and often, it is their only job. If they choose to do their only job poorly, why are they kept on the payroll? Please, every manager who reads this, either bring these employees to your level of expectations or let them go.

I was recently told by a newly hired chef that we "always compromise down." Many managers just give in because it is easier to compromise than it is to uphold standards.

This hit me like a ton of bricks. He was so right. Hospital culture is so different from restaurant culture. Most hospitals have very generous vacation policies and very liberal employee health programs—any employee who really wants a weekend off can go and make up some ridiculous aliment and get time off. This is unheard of in the restaurant world. Can you imagine working in a restaurant and going to some health clinic that gives the employee a note saying because their head or back hurts that you not only have to give them four days off, you have to pay them for it? That is what we deal with. The employees know it, and they use it to their advantage all the time.

Firing employees is the hardest task any manager has to do. I know from experience that if we do not get the best employees working for us, we will never achieve what we are trying to do. However, firing people should be the last resort. Most employees, when given the right encouragement and the right training, will usually rise to the occasion. I have found over the years that it is better to spend time with them, find out what they need, and give them the tools that they need to be successful. This usually works, but you do have some employees who just don't get it. To these employees, there is only one choice: you must show them the door. Your parting thoughts should be, "I hope they go work for the competitor. They will do great. Good luck and good-bye."

The Tray Line

Most of you have never witnessed this spectacular event; it is like controlled chaos. An outsider could never imagine exactly what is going on. We recently had a photographer from a Raleigh newspaper do a story on us. He said that he had covered some interesting things over his career, but he had never witnessed the intensity of feeding 350 people at once. He told me that what he saw was amazing, I said that was not amazing, that was lunch. We do this three times a day, 365 days a year.

In hospitals, tray lines are configured in many ways. Some are more modern, some are very old. Some are modeled for room service—much like a hotel—and some are modeled in a traditional manner; i.e., all the patients get mostly the same thing and the trays just move around the belt.

Most tray lines are mechanical—a motorized belt pushes trays along much like an automobile assembly line works. The employees work at the speed of the belt. There are some hospitals that just have a set of rollers where you manually roll the trays down the line. Either way, the goal is to move the tray to another position so that the next employee can add what they need to the tray.

The "Starter"

The first position is called the "starter." This person begins the process of setting up the trays for each patient. The food is served on a very hot plate and put onto what is called a *pellet.* This pellet is then placed on a piece of equipment called an "activator" that heats it. The pellet will stay hot for approximately forty-five minutes. Once the food is put on plates, it is covered with a dome lid, which is insulated to help keep the food hot. It is not the sexiest way to serve food, but it does the job.

In a traditional tray line, the starter sets the first tray down on the belt and adds the silverware, napkin, the condiments, and the menu itself. These menus are often filled out by the patient the day before. If the patient does not fill out a menu, a meal is preselected for them and sent down the line. Every hospital is different and may not do this exactly the same way we do, but the end result is the same—the food begins to move down the line. The starter will also look at the diet that is prescribed to the patient. If the patient is a diabetic, an artificial sweetener will be added instead of sugar; a salt alternative is included for heart-healthy and low-sodium diets, etc. The starters control the pace and are usually the most experienced employees working on that shift.

The Disher

In a traditional tray line, the dishers will look at the ticket and add the appropriate menu items to the activated pellet/plate. They *dish* out the hot entree, sauces, vegetable, and starch onto the plate per the patient's order and diet restrictions. Then they pass it to the next person on the line.

The "Next Person"

The next person will add the rest of the items. The belt goes around and multiple employees will add the remaining items on the menu—salads, dressings, desserts, beverages, fruit, and anything else the patient wants. The tray continues around until it gets to the checker

The Checker

This person is usually a senior employee. They look at the tray and make sure that all the items requested are on it. They set the completed trays into carts and push them over to the Patient Services team. These folks are called many different things in various hospitals. I have heard them called catering associates, room service attendants, patient-service employees, and the like. Their jobs are all the same—get the food to the patient as quickly as possible. This is the hard part.

The Workstation Method

Some contract companies and self-operated hospitals have transitioned the traditional tray lines into *workstations*. This is where the employee who serves the food will actually build the trays, customized to each individual patient. This is much better than a tray line. The rationale is that the person who serves the food and builds the tray will be more cognizant of the patient's needs; they have met the patient and have taken their order. This system is almost like room service. The server can offer suggestions, read and explain the menu, and help the patient get what they want. It is very effective, and most hospitals are turning this way.

The hospital at which I currently work has actual room service, just like a hotel. The patient reads a menu, orders from the phone, and within an hour, the food is delivered by one of our employees. This is the ideal way to serve food. The patient gets what they want when they want, and they feel special. It also saves a lot of money in food cost. Many patients eat light and may only want a bowl of soup and a small salad. If you send up a tray of grilled salmon with brown rice and roasted asparagus, they may not eat it, and it just gets thrown away. Patients who get what they want are happier patients, and happy patients give us better scores on our surveys, and that is the key.

The Delivery

The carts are loaded according to floor and sent to specific areas in the hospital. The employee pushes the carts to the appropriate room and serves the food to the patients. This is the part that often gets overlooked when troubleshooting problems. There are so many things that can happen between the kitchen and the patients.

Elevators

All hospitals have them, and if you are not fortunate enough to have your own elevators dedicated to the kitchen, then you could be in for a long, drawn-out journey. Elevators in hospitals are very busy. I have seen room service attendants wait ten minutes for an elevator, only to have it full of people and have to wait some more. The cargo elevators can also be full with vast amounts of equipment and supplies that are constantly being delivered throughout the hospital. It can be frustrating just getting the food upstairs. This gets even harder when an elevator is down for service.

Socializing

I am talking about the employee who has to socialize with everyone they see in the hallway. Most hospital employees have been on the job for many years—my current staff averages about nine years. The food service people know everyone in every department and often feel they must stop and talk to them. I have found employees actually sitting in lobbies with their carts talking to people. I have seen some standing at nurses' stations eating candy, drinking soda, and basically just wasting precious time. They are doing everything but serving the patients their food. Meanwhile, the food is getting cold.

Cell Phones

If workers are not talking to someone in the hallway, they are talking on the phone. This drives me crazy. I think the world was a better place when we did not have cell phones. They are disruptive and annoying. Just the other day, I found one of our room-service attendants sitting on a bench, outside an elevator, talking on her cell phone with a full cart of patient food. When she saw me, she hung up on the person and quickly began pushing her cart down the hall. I told her that cell phone usage was against policy in the hospital. Her response was that it was her kid. This, of course, is the standard reply that we get. They think it gets them off the hook. What they do not realize is that cell phones can interfere with patient monitoring equipment and can actually put the patient at harm. Plus, my food is getting cold. Get off the damn phone!

The Nursing Station

If a patient is in an isolation room, the food service employee may not be allowed to enter the patient's room. This varies from hospital to hospital. If they are not allowed in, they drop the food off at the nurses' station. It then begins to die a slow death. The nurses are very busy people. They sometimes look at food as a burden or an inconvenience. Sometimes they don't even see it at all. It is only when the patient begins to complain that they take notice.

I can't tell you how many times I have seen our trays just sitting there at the nurses' station. The coffee is cold, the milk is warm, the food is cold, and all of our hard work is ruined. Most importantly, the food may have become unsafe. If food sits in the danger zone too long, harmful bacteria can begin to grow. This is the last thing we want to happen to a patient who is in an isolation room due to a weakened immune system. It could be fatal.

Of course, the end result is always our fault. After the patient complains that the food is cold, Nursing will tell the patient, "Yeah, those Food and Nutrition people just don't get it." The nurses will often go and microwave the food, which makes it even worse. The food was hot, it was served on time, but it sat there and died.

I have battled this for years and I have never been able to get it fixed. I have asked Nursing to call us, so that we can send a new tray. I would rather throw the food away than serve an unsafe, poor quality tray to a patient.

The Patient Test

The other part of our cold food problem has to do with the tests that patients receive as part of their treatment. In a traditional tray line, the food is sent up at a specific time. Many patients are constantly being removed from their rooms and taken to other areas of the hospital. They get x-rays, MRIs, surgeries, etc. Often they do not come back for quite awhile.

If the food is put in the room, it could be hours before they get to eat it. So, we are back to the cold food problem again. There is no way for the people in Food and Nutrition to know if a patient is getting tested or what time they will be back. The solution is communication from Nursing, (which happens infrequently) or to have room service in your hospital, where the food is not delivered until the patient calls. This is really quite elementary.

Still-Missing Items on the Trays

Over and over again we heard from our patients that items were missing on their trays. This problem was still rearing its ugly head: the patients were not getting what they ordered. In a traditional tray line, the patients get a menu the day prior to the meal. They fill it out and hand it back to the nurses or to someone in Food and Nutrition. These orders are taken to our diet office, and they are entered into our computer software program that spits out a ticket for the tray-line employees.

Part of the problem lies with ordering the food a day ahead of time. Most patients cannot remember what they ordered twenty-four hours ago. What seemed good then may not be what they want to eat now. Patients are sick and have good days and bad days. Hospitals need to get the patients to order the day *of* the meal, instead of the day prior. Many problems could be solved with this approach. But I had a feeling that the bigger part lay somewhere else.

We had fixed our problems with bad food for the most part, but patients were still not getting everything they ordered. I began to dig into this. *Why were so many patients still saying the same thing?* We were paying someone to look at the trays and ensure that patients got what they ordered. That is all they had to do. What was the problem? How is it the Checker position failed repeatedly?

I met with my checkers and asked them. They insisted they'd put everything on the tray that the patient requested. They read the tickets just as it was written and did exactly that. They could not figure out why the problem existed either. Neither of us could.

Then, I had one of my many epiphanies. I went to a local restaurant for breakfast one day with my wife and son. We sat down and ordered our food. When the food arrived, I looked at my plate. I had a cup of coffee, pancakes, eggs, bacon, biscuits, and fresh fruit. I looked around the table and noticed that the waitress had brought cream and sugar for my coffee, syrup and butter for my pancakes, and jelly for my biscuits. She even asked if I wanted hot sauce for my eggs. Well, you know I actually did, so I said, "Yes, I would like hot sauce for my eggs."

I thought to myself, *I never asked for these. They just came.* It is what is expected with food. When was the last time you ordered pancakes at a restaurant and said, "Oh, by the way, can I have some syrup with those pancakes?" You never do; you just assume that it will be there. Maybe this was our problem. Maybe patients just assumed that certain items would be on the tray without having to order them. I began to look into this.

I asked the diet-office employees to begin to track the items that patients said were missing on the trays. Creamers, coffee, sugar, syrup, and butter were on the top of the list. I had my clinical manager at Rex Health Care do the same, and the results were not as dramatic—but Rex uses room service, so our employees speak with the patients as they order their food. That staff was trained to ask the right questions: "Do you want creamer with your coffee? Do you want coffee? How about syrup with those pancakes?" It was such a difference when I ran the same test against a traditional tray-line setting. We were missing *all* of these items. The mindset of most hospital food service workers is if they don't order it, they don't get it. It's almost like the cost of the food is coming out of their pockets. Give them the creamer!

The patients, on the other hand, just assumed that many of these items would be there. It was a revelation, and we began to fix it. But once again, I ran into the dietitian roadblock.

The dietitians said that adding sugar, creamer, jelly, syrup, etc. would throw off the balance of the amount of carbohydrates the patient was receiving. My response was, "Let's take pancakes, French toast, coffee, and biscuits off the menu then." If we continued to serve these without normal condiments, then we would continue to get bad scores. We also had sugar-free alternatives to all of our condiments. There should be no reason these were not served. Pancakes should be served with syrup and mashed potatoes should be served with gravy. Coffee should be served with cream and sugar, or at least a sugar substitute.

I argued a good case, and I got my way. The only stipulation was allergies. If a patient had a gluten allergy, they could not have gravy. This made sense to me. I did not want to hurt the patient. I just wanted good food served.

So, we began to add condiments to the trays, and the scores went up. The bottom line is, if you serve food that is prepared correctly, get it to the patient quickly, and give them what they want, you will have better scores. It is simple. I had fought for years to get to this point, and it was finally working.

The hospitals that are serving food that patients do not want will never achieve what they are trying to do. I believe that this is the biggest problem hospitals face. There is so much food being prepared for patients that they do not order themselves. I see it all the time. I used to run percentages on each floor of how many patients order. The floors that had low percentages of patient-ordered food had lower scores. It was amazing to me that in all the years that I worked for mega contractors no one ever figured it out. I knew this from personal experience. I was on the receiving end once, and I never forgot it.

In 1986, I was at Fort Benning, going through Airborne training. I had just lost my long-time girlfriend, whom I loved very much, via a "Dear John" letter.[6] I was far away from my friends and family, and I wanted to go home. Airborne training was tough. The Black Hats were relentless, and I was surviving day by day.

Our company was marched to chow one day during the training. We would run six abreast up the stairs and get in line. There were hundreds of troopers trying to get food. We would only get thirty minutes to eat.

6 This is the letter that all GI's hope they never get. It is a letter saying that the girlfriend or wife they had when they went into the service has decided that she will not wait while they are serving their country. In other words, they have moved on to another guy. Painful!

These thirty minutes started when the first person got in the door. If you were last or near the end, you often had to get your food and eat as much as you could as you walked to the tray return. Time was up, and you had no time to even sit down. It was intense.

One particular day at breakfast, I was starving and at the end of the line. I had eaten my meal on the way to the trashcan; our thirty minutes were up, and I had just gotten my plate. But it was time to go. As I was leaving the mess hall, I was dreaming about eggs, bacon, toast, and anything else I could get, but I had to slide it into the trash or risk being singled out for a day of living hell.

Later during that day I had run miles, did thousands of pushups, got yelled at all day, and burned many calories. I was tired and wanted to eat. I was looking forward to eating some chow. When I got to the serving line at the dinner meal, I was given a plate with baked cod, cauliflower, and rice. I told the cook that I didn't like fish and asked if I could have another option. Well, the Black Hat who was standing beside me went ballistic in the typical Airborne instructor fashion. He was yelling and screaming at me, telling me I was lucky to get anything and to get the hell off his chow line. I took my tray and quickly got as far away from him as I could. I sat down and almost lost it. I had been through so much. I was in one of the toughest training schools the army had to offer. I was handling it well; I could do all that they wanted: I ran. I did pushups. I jumped from towers. I was keeping up with the rest of the students. I was doing things I never would have dreamed of. I said to myself daily, "I can take anything they dish out, I will do this. I can handle it."

What I could not handle was the food I had in front of me. I still remember that meal, twenty-plus years later. I remember how that meal almost broke me. I was so hungry that I was forced to eat it. It was awful. It was the worst meal I had ever had. I was so upset, I wanted to go AWOL and just go home. I remember saying, "That's it, they won. I am done with this crap." I was prepared for the penalty; I wanted to go home. I wanted to quit.

Well, quitting and going on the run from the military police was not in my nature. I never could have lived with myself and could never have looked into my father's eyes again. So I pulled up my bootstraps, stopped feeling sorry for myself, and went back to work.

However, I have never forgotten that day. It was the worst day I had ever had in the army. It was not the Airborne training. It was not the runs. It was not the physical training. It was not the Black Hats. It was not even the fact that my girlfriend had dumped me via the US Mail. It was the cod! It was the freakin' cod that broke me.

I realize today that this is how my patients were feeling. I once had a patient who told me she could never eat enchiladas again. We serve a vegetarian black bean enchilada on our menu. This patient was one of the many who did not order her food, so a meal was automatically sent to her. Well, the meal she got was our enchilada. She was recovering from cancer treatments and felt very nauseous. When the food arrived, she lifted up the lid and immediately threw up. She told me later that she could never eat another enchilada again for the rest of her life. In fact, she said we had ruined it for her.

This is a great example of what happens when you just send food to a patient that they are not expecting. These people are sick and very sensitive to various foods, aromas, and tastes. If we had just allowed her to choose what she wanted to eat, she would have been happy. Maybe she wanted a bowl of soup and crackers, or maybe a grilled cheese. We failed to give her what she wanted, and she became sick because of it. Plus, for all our pain and her dissatisfaction, it added additional cost, as we had to replace the tray we already sent with what she really wanted. It was a lose-lose situation, and hospitals all around the country still do this over and over again every day.

She had had the codfish meal that I had many years ago. She will remember that meal forever, just as I have.

The Culture of Health Care

Action expresses priority.

—Mohandas Gandhi

The culture that is ingrained in any health-care setting is unlike any other business setting. It is unique in so many ways and on so many levels. Food service in health care is the last of the great frontiers. Restaurants, hotels, food courts, and colleges have risen to the calls of their customers. Most hospitals have not risen to that call. It is an environment of entitlement and is not now, nor will be for a long time, an environment of change.

Restaurants have adapted their menus to attract customers. They offer value meals, discounts, or two for $19.99 at many of the big chains. Some of the great big restaurant chefs have adapted. They have created airport venues that offer fantastic bistro-style food at affordable prices for travelers. Wolfgang Puck created the California-style pizza that is available in any supermarket. Chefs and restaurant owners, in a battle for survival, must adapt and change to their customers' needs and must be willing to take a risk.

The days of the long, drawn-out, very expensive meal at restaurants are not as popular as they once were. There are of course very high-end restaurants that cater to a group of people who spend big money on food. However I feel that most of America is looking for something quick and affordable. I do believe that Americans still want quality food and are willing to pay for it, but it has to be reasonable. I think that owning a restaurant in 2010 must be the hardest thing. People are just more conscious of what they spend. Restaurant owners know this and adapt accordingly.

Hotels have seen hard times as well. Traveling Americans are not as abundant as they once were. I remember spending many nights in hotels throughout Washington, DC, and in almost every hotel I stayed at, they closed their restaurants due to low patronage. These were decent hotels, as the company I was working for paid the bill. I would not stay at anything less than a Marriott Courtyard.

The hotel I stayed at frequently was on Embassy Row in DC. It was a hotel located right across the street from a few embassies. It was a very nice part of DC, located near Seventeenth street. It had a full-service restaurant and bar. I stayed there for almost two months, and within those two months, I saw the restaurant close and re-open with a trendy "take-out bistro" menu, attracting the people walking by from the Metro station at DuPont Circle. They had adapted to their environment, and they had survived. They only survived by change. Change is necessary in our world; without change, you simply go out of business.

Colleges were among the first to adapt. The mall generation of kids who grew up going to malls and eating at various national and regional brands made this happen. The food courts of the late eighties and early nineties were relatively new, and they were a big draw on the youth of America. The malls provided quick, trendy food that was appealing to seventeen/eighteen year olds. These brands, for the most part, had the marketing—the TV commercials—and they had America's teenagers standing in line to spend their parents' dollars at their restaurants. Have you ever eaten at one of these "great burger" places, or the chicken place with two pickles and a soft hamburger roll? The food sucked, but the kids loved it, and the money came pouring in. These companies had marketed to the audience they were serving, and they made an impression. What they were doing was the expected norm; it was not good food, but it was what sold, and these companies were riding the wave. The food was mediocre, but well displayed and well marketed and was what these kids wanted.

Then these high school teenagers went to college. It was all about to change. Contract companies are the first to adapt to change. They have teams of people who sit around tables and think up stuff—they video conference with each other around the country, just thinking up new programs and concepts. They want to keep their contracts, and they know students who are unhappy with the food being served can get them thrown off campus. That was the last thing anyone wanted, and they did whatever it took to stay there. Money means success and success is what drives careers. They had to change. I worked in colleges from 1992–2002, and I saw it all happen, right before my eyes.

I remember visiting Green Mountain College in Poultney, Vermont, while on vacation. A good friend of mine was going there, and I went to see her. The company that ran the food service did an awful job. Even in my hung-over state, desperately needing food, I could not eat it. This was 1987. Years later, when I worked in colleges, I thought to myself, "Wow, college food service has certainly grown up."

These kids coming into college expected more. They had seen the food courts in the malls, and they wanted *that* food. We had to adjust to their needs. We adapted our menus to fit their appetites. We made food that they wanted; we did what the malls were doing. We had them trapped, and our goal was to take as much money out of their pockets as we could. If anyone says otherwise, they are lying.

Sales were everything to us. It was our lifeblood. Late-night pizza study breaks, smoothies and milk shakes, vegan food, free Tibet, save the whales, save the Earth … We did whatever they wanted. I once bought an $11,000-Styrofoam *densifier* that we used to recycle Styrofoam, because a group of students wanted it. It was all about the contract. We made a fortune off those students.

College food progressed by this catalyst called money. Today's universities offer incredible food, at least compared to college food service back in the 80s. They have barbecue concepts where they smoke their own briskets and pork butts. They make pizza dough from scratch. They cook food correctly. They have sushi made onsite. They do theme meals and hire chefs to make their food better. It's all about the dollar. If they do not provide this, the students will go somewhere else. It is that simple—supply and demand.

There are colleges that make their own cheese and have sustainable farms that provide their produce. There is a college in Massachusetts that hosts an annual chefs' conference to bring college chefs from around the country to help develop skills they can take back to make their food better. College food service has indeed come a long way. It is truly a mega-million-dollar business. Colleges are the golden goose for contractors. They listen to their customers, and they react accordingly.

Health care is a different story. The employees in the health-care industry for the most part are hard working, good, honest people. I have met many over the years whom I consider good friends. The problem is that the culture has not adapted to the ever-changing world of food service.

Hospitals are in the business of health care. Their primary mission is to take care of the well-being of their patients. It is often a world where very little money is being invested in food service. The primary mission is to invest in new technology, obtain the best doctors, and expand treatment for the sick and injured. When I worked at my second hospital in DC, they installed a new Gamma Knife that could do surgery on brain disorders using radiation. The result was that the patient could be treated by a dose of gamma radiation right to the source of the problem. Pretty amazing stuff. This is where hospitals spend their capital. I know that this is important, and it is where they should spend their money, but if they want good food, they must siphon a little off to the Food and Nutrition department.

Additionally, many employees in the health-care industry possess an entitlement mentality. Hospitals are the last institutions to still offer the kind of benefits that most small business and even corporate employees would dream of. At UNCH, starting employees receive seven weeks of paid time off per year. Seven weeks! When I worked for contract companies, we had two vacation weeks, and if you worked there for five years, you would get three weeks. That is how it should be. The amount of time off in health-care settings is disruptive, and I know it will be looked at in the coming years as health-care costs continue to rise.

When management has to decline a request for vacation time, we hear from our employees that it is their "right" to have time off and we cannot deny it. This is absurd—we can deny time off. We are at the mercy of our patients, not our staff. Patient care comes first. I am not saying that we enjoy denying vacation; of course we don't. We want our employees to take time off with their families. Quality of life is important, but we also have a job to do.

Some of the things that really bother me about health care that are unheard of in other industries are as follows:

Free Food

Hospitals often reward employees for a job well done. This may be due to a successful hospital accreditation survey, to celebrate high patient satisfaction, or just simply to celebrate the holidays. Hospitals are well known for free meals at Thanksgiving and Christmas. I agree that we should celebrate success; it makes the employees feel appreciated, and it is the right thing to do.

However, in all my years of doing this, I have only seen the ugly side of humanity. It is a travesty of poor behavior I have actually seen people push each other to get more of the free food. It reminds me of that poor guy who died at a Wal-Mart on the first day of the Christmas shopping season. He was trampled to death over a PlayStation, or a Wii, or whatever sale they had that day. It was a disgrace and everyone involved in his death should spend the rest of their lives in prison. It was horrible to watch. That is what it is like when you yell "free food" in a hospital; people will come running.

Ice Cream Socials

I specifically remember one incident. We had received no deficiencies on our Joint Commission survey and this was a big deal, so the administration wanted to celebrate. They called us and arranged a free ice cream social for five thousand employees. This ice cream social included all the toppings to make sundaes. We ordered all of the ingredients, and we set the tables up for service.

We had to have hospital police there, because a crowd was forming. They had formed a line one hour before we actually opened. These people were standing in line waiting for free ice cream. It was hard to believe. My question as a manager was, how did they have an hour to wait in line? They should have been at their jobs taking care of patients, or if they were not directly involved with patient care, they should have been helping those who were. Weren't they supposed to be working? I could not believe what was going on.

When we actually opened, it was a mob scene. There were people pushing each other, yelling, cursing at each other. I was appalled at the behavior that was taking place in front of me. I was standing at the door allowing only a few at a time into the room where the ice cream was. One lady came out with a plate of ice cream that was the biggest portion of ice cream I have ever seen. I had had enough. I stopped her and asked, "How on earth can anyone eat that much ice cream?" It looked like the box you buy at the grocery store; you know, the rectangle box that you scoop from. And it was covered with whipped cream, cherries, chocolate, the works.

Her response was, "I'm gonna get what is mine." I was floored! I could not believe that people were behaving this way over free ice cream. I went home that day very sad at what I had observed. It was amazing—all over free ice cream. I wanted nothing to do with this ever gain. It was embarrassing. It was shameful. I can almost understand how police officers get out of hand. They see the worst of society—I certainly had! If I'd had a Taser gun that day, I would have used it. I really felt like sending in tear gas and disbursing the crowd, but I probably would have had a problem with Human Resources. So reluctantly, I had to restrain myself.

Holiday Meals

This is another big problem for the people who provide food to hospitals. Over the years, I have heard from health-care workers that it is their "right" to free food on the holidays. Now, I have read the Constitution and the Declaration of Independence many times. If you never have, you should. They really blast King George, and it was ambitious for a bunch of colonialists to take this dramatic stand against the strongest military power on earth. I love it. These people were pretty brave. They were the rock stars of the day.

The problem is that every time I read it, I never have seen that free food on holidays is an inalienable right. I do see the freedom of speech, the right to face your accuser, the right to a trial by your peers, and the right to bear arms is all there. Nowhere in those documents does it say that health-care workers will get a free meal on holidays. So stop this nonsense. The reason you are getting a free meal is that the hospital administration where you work is paying for it. So behave yourself and be thankful that they see the value in supplying a meal for you.

Employee Discounts

The Holy Grail of health-care employee entitlements is the employee discount. This is another "right" I have never been able to find. However, I hear time and time again that it is a right. I have worked in two hospitals that did not offer an employee discount, and the employees survived. I hear over and over again from employees, "Why are your prices so high?" or "We can't afford this." I even hear that "us poor people" can't afford it.

I spent some time in Panama, Honduras, and El Salvador. The people that I met in those countries were truly poor. So, when you say that you are poor and that you cannot afford your five-dollar meal—please consider what a meal at any local restaurant would cost. I bet it is more than five dollars. The poor people in those Central American countries are truly poor. Many have no running water, no electricity, and minimal (if any) medical attention. When I hear the term *poor people,* I think of those folks. I recently watched a video of Michelle Obama serving food in a homeless shelter in DC. The camera that was filming it recorded many people standing in line taking pictures of her on their cell phones. The people I saw standing in line for food in South America most definitely did not have cell phones. How can you be homeless and have a cell phone? Where do they send the bill? That is another story for another day.

I offer a "5 for 5" menu special. This means that you get an entree, two sides, a roll, and a beverage for $5.00, including tax. These entrees include a choice of chicken satay, braised lamb shanks, grilled pork chops, ribs, half-roasted chicken, and Louisiana jambalaya. The main dishes are served with your choice of sides, a fresh baked roll, and a beverage. You cannot go to McDonald's and get a meal for that price. The last time I looked, McDonald's was not serving braised lamb shanks and grilled rib-eye steaks with sautéed mushrooms and onions. If you find a place that offers the same quality food for the mere price of $5.00 let me know. I want to go.

I do know that spending five to six dollars a day gets expensive; I had to do it for three months and I hated it. However, whenever I went outside the café, it always cost me more. Restaurants in town are always more expensive than ours is.

The idea that because you work in a hospital environment your food should be free or subsidized is an idea of days gone by. Companies can no longer afford to subsidize employee meals. It is the reality of our time. Those days are over. It costs money to serve you and all we are asking is that you pay what is fair. A grilled salmon with two sides and a drink would cost you over $15 in any restaurant. We serve it all-inclusive for $5.00, including tax.

Rex Health Care

The bus came by and I got on; that's when it all began.

—Jerry Garcia

In the fall of 2008, while I was working at UNCH, the administration at Rex decided to make a change with its food service department. It was being run by one of the mega contractors, and change was needed. They asked me to be the director and take over the operations. We had built an empire at UNCH. Our food was good; our programs were sound; and we knew that we could easily move these programs into Rex without any problems.

Angelo Mojica and I packed up our bag of tricks and headed to Raleigh. Angelo's job was to help with the two nursing homes that came with the package. He had experience in that area, while I had never even been in a nursing home; so I let him handle that one. Nursing homes are a completely different world of food service—the final insult in the food service world—and we all need to really put some effort into the quality of food in these places. It is beyond sad.

We had three months to plan and build a team. I got busy writing menus, hiring my management team, and observing the outgoing contractor. I wanted this to be different, so I took the time to plan and work the menus to be the best you could find in any hospital in North Carolina. I wanted a great heart-healthy and low-sodium menu, and I took much of what I did at UNCH to develop this one. The difference now was I had room service; I wanted the food to be memorable.

As the time for transition was approaching fast, my new managers and I had to get things in gear. The contractor was still there, so we could not get into the kitchen like we wanted to. We had no storage place for our food, nor were we allowed to train the staff. They were on the job producing the contractor's menu, and pulling them off to train on our new menu was impossible. It was going to be a rough opening. One week before our opening, we rented two refrigerated semi-trucks from our food distributor. The refrigerated trucks were full with our new menu items sitting on the loading dock. My new chef had gone a little crazy and ordered enough food to feed a small nation. I have to admit, I was a little annoyed. It took us two days to unload those trucks. In his defense, he was new to Rex and new to the menu. He erred in having too much, which is preferable to having too little.

On January 13, 2009, at the stroke of midnight, we transitioned the management from a contractor to a self-operated facility. We were all there and began moving equipment and setting up for our first meal, just hours away.

I must say, the contractors who were leaving were very honorable in the transition of management. I have seen others damage operations by not forwarding pre-booked caterings or disabling the registers. I have even seen one contractor break equipment, remove coffee urns, and remove property that was not theirs. This management group did the opposite. They did not like the fact that they were getting the boot, but they went out with dignity. The director treated me with courtesy and gave me as much information as he could. The patient service manager even worked diligently on getting our employee vacancies filled before she left. I had a lot of respect for this team; they could have been much worse than they were. They were a group of folks that I would have loved to have a beer with—but I was the one taking their jobs, so beer was not the order of the day.

Meanwhile, we had not spent one moment training the cooks and other employees on what to do. We had to do it on the run, and that is what we did.

Our first breakfast went really well in our retail operations. The food was great. We had many new menu items that the employees at Rex had never seen in the café. We did grilled pineapple, fried pork chops, hash-brown casseroles, and a variety of omelets and fresh-made eggs. We had a display selection of fresh fruit and yogurt and a variety of grab-and-go sandwiches. The lines looked great and the food was well prepared and well displayed.

Our patient food was another story. The food was great, but we were way behind on the tray line. We had massive computer problems that caused major issues. It was really painful. We had our Information Technology people all day with us trying to fix it. The company that sold us the software sent a representative to help us, but she just got in the way. During our most difficult time in getting the lunch meal out, I found her eating in the office completely oblivious to our problems. It was a terrible morning to say the least. I called her company and told them that she was no longer welcome at Rex. She was supposed to be there to help, but instead she did nothing. Admittedly, she may not have caused our problems, but she could have prevented many of them if she had done what she was paid to do.

We eventually worked it out and did a decent dinner. The food was beginning to go out on time, and the cooks were submitting to intense training on the fly throughout the day. They were so used to scooping overcooked, bland, institutional food, and now, we were cooking our food to order. If the ticket from the printer said, "Lime and ginger–glazed salmon," we pulled a piece of salmon out of the marinade and placed it on the grill. We were running like a restaurant; our food was fresh and being cooked as food should be—with lots of love. It was amazing to see the tickets go out. We had had such a bad morning, but by 6:00 PM, the food was looking good, and the staff was beginning to get more comfortable. It was a rough day, but we made it through.

Every day after that day, we got better. Our food was good and our patients were seeing the change. The most impressive statements were from the patients who were there during the transformation. They had received dinner from the contractor, and then for the next meal at breakfast, they got our food. The comments we received were great—with only the negative comment that the food took forever to arrive. We definitely had work to do.

The next few weeks were rough; we had to stabilize the madness that was our kitchen. We had so much to do. It was going to be a long, arduous task, but I had a good staff and a great management team. We would overcome this.

That first day, we had people from all over the hospital helping us get the food out. We even had some vice presidents running food. It was good to see that Rex was a hospital that looked at things differently. They knew that when one department fails, they all fail. It is a very different place, one that truly cares about outcomes and is keenly aware of just how intertwined each department is. Failure was not an option on January 14, 2009.

Within a few days, we had it running somewhat smoothly, and the compliments were coming in. Even so, it was extremely painful; probably the hardest opening I ever went through. Without the dedication of my team, we would have never made it.

Working at Rex has changed my life for the better. I have been able to drive our program with full support of the administration. The people that I work with truly care about what they do, and it shows in their faces that they are glad to be there. We have a saying at Rex that we are "chosen for excellence." This is more than a slogan; our co-workers truly live by this motto. They know that how we interact with patients and visitors will have a huge impact on their decision-making when it comes to choosing health-care providers. We in Food and Nutrition hope they come for the food, but humbly have to admit they are coming to Rex because of the excellent medical care they receive. Though great food doesn't hurt.

Rex was voted in 2009 as one of the best places to work by *Modern Healthcare* magazine, and it was recognized as a Thomson Reuters 100 Top Hospitals national award winner—the only hospital in North Carolina to receive this award.

The Software That Makes Patient-Feeding Possible

We've got to put a lot of money into changing behavior.

—Bill Gates, Microsoft

I had developed the new menu and written all of the recipes, but now I had to enter them into the software program that would run our patient-feeding process. This software allows patients' preferences to be entered into the database. All of this is done item by item. Every ingredient has to be entered—salt, pepper, onions, celery—anything and everything that is in the recipe has to be entered one by one. There were thousands of items that had to be entered. It was a grueling task. Luckily, I had help from some really good employees who did most of the groundwork. My job was to write and enter the recipes—one-by-painful-one. It took me almost three months to get it done

Once it's done, however, the software can do some amazing things. Many people do not realize how much goes into this. You pick up the phone or circle your menu, and you think, "That's it. That was pretty easy." It is not so easy. It is very complicated and a lot of effort from many people goes into delivering your soup to your room.

The most complex part is the way food is run through the system of ordering. The software will provide the correct nutrition information for the correct patient. It takes into consideration allergies and carbohydrates, as well as likes and dislikes, and more.

For example, Mr. Jones is admitted to the hospital. He is a diabetic and is allergic to seafood. He does not like onions and prefers decaf to regular coffee. The nurses on the floor will enter this information into the database. When the patient orders the food (in our case, they order by phone), our staff will open that patient's file and take the order.

If Mr. Jones tries to order too many carbohydrates, the system will not allow it. The person on the phone will direct him to order something else. The software will also search the entire recipe database and find any menu item that may have seafood in it. If he tried to order something that had some sort of seafood ingredient, it will also block the order.

The software also finds recipes that contain onions, and the patient will again be directed to another choice. It will also list the patient's preference to decaf coffee. It is pretty amazing how it works, despite how painful it is to input all the background data.

This software is very complicated and does not always work. The restrictions that the system puts on certain diets are a good thing, but it can also be bad. In a traditional hospital setting, patients order the food in advance. Orders are usually taken from menus that are handed out to the patients. The patients then choose what they want and hand it back. As usual, the problem is with patients who have meals automatically sent.

When the patient does not order, the software will create a menu for them. It does not rationalize. It does not think about what is good or how that meal may look on the plate. All it does is search for allergies, the type of diet the patient is on, and what preferences they have. This can produce horrible results. We once had thirty patients get a hardboiled egg as their dinner meal.

It's not just the software's fault when something like this happens. The worst part was that no one on the tray line thought to question it. These hard-boiled egg meals probably passed by twenty people before the patients received them, and no one said anything. I found out by the multiple patient complaints we received! It was pretty embarrassing. This only strengthened my point about making sure patients fill out their orders—and that we needed people to actually think about what they were doing. The computer should only be a tool, not the ultimate decision maker.

Room Service

After all the years of looking at retherm, cook/chill food, and at food coming off traditional tray lines, I finally had the grand prize in heath care food service. I had room service. This is by far the best way to serve food in a hospital. The patients simply pick up the phone after looking at the menu located in their room, and place their order. Our menu looks exactly like what you would see in a hotel with room service and is just as good.

The room service call center person receives the call and enters the patient's food order into the system. Once all the restrictions have been met, the computer forwards it to our kitchen printers. These printers are the same as any you would find in any restaurant. Once the ticket prints, the cooks rip it off the printer, and place it on their line.

The idea is that once the tickets are printed, we would have the food in the patient's room freshly cooked, piping hot, and delicious. Sounds pretty easy, right? Well it most definitely is not easy. In fact, it is probably the hardest thing in the world. And indeed painful at times. Our problem was that the cooks were still hospital cooks. They were not fast-moving restaurant cooks. They saw things very differently from how a restaurant cook would. I have to hand it to them though; after a few months they did rise to the occasion and (for the most part) became a pretty strong group. For one, they are cooking the food better—they actually taste the food they cook! Something they never did before. But most important, they are beginning to care. Each one of them had it in them; they just needed someone to help them find their way. At the writing of this book, we have taken our patient satisfaction scores from 22 percent to 94, in the excellent range. This is huge for any hospital setting, and it was huge for us.

Our patients can choose from our Chef-Inspired menu items, which might include pecan-crusted chicken served with a maple butter sauce. They can have grilled flank steak with an ancho chili and grilled corn salsa. They can order handmade vegetarian lasagna with squash and portabella mushrooms, served in a creamy Alfredo sauce.

We also have Comfort Favorites, such as country-style meatloaf, herb-crusted chicken, or Carolina pulled-pork barbecue. They can also order "From the Grill" with items such as burgers, cheese-steaks, grilled-cheese sandwiches, and so on. We also offer a variety of salads, handmade desserts, and a list of fresh-made side dishes.

The beauty of room service is that we don't cook your meal until you order it. Things like meatloaf, lasagna, and roasted turkey are cooked ahead of time and served in portions like any restaurant would, but items such as fajitas, shish kabob, grilled pork chops, flank steak, etc. are cooked to order. The result is the restaurant-quality food I had been searching for.

I had made the long journey for good food in hospitals, and I believe we have achieved that goal.

The ultimate quest is still not over. We will continue to refine our program, rewriting the menus to reflect the seasons and training our cooks in our *Black Hat Chef* program. We will continue to raise the bar.

What's Next?

How come my priority list is horizontal?

—Paul Berens, my business manager at Rex talking about my never-ending new ideas, which usually results in his doing more work.

It has taken a lot of hard work to achieve what I did these past years. I had to be a mentor, disciplinarian, and chef. I had to put up with terminations, unemployment hearings, and long counseling sessions. I had to take on the unions. I had to take on the dietitians and the nurses. I had to plead my case wherever and to whomever I could. I had to get around rules or just plain break them. I even had to leave a company I truly loved in the quest for good food. I had to sit on the line for hundreds of hours just to ensure the food was right, sending food back when it was not—always an act of endearment to my cooks. In the beginning, they looked at me as a jerk—always complaining about the food. The fact was, it was never personal; it was always about the food.

I recently had a conversation with one of my cooks who had been at Rex for many years and had gone through many changes. He said that he'd "figured me out," explaining that "if you want Jim to go away, just do what is expected. Cook the food correctly, serve it hot, serve it quick, and serve it with love." He said that he'd told his fellow cooks, "Jim only wants good food. If you take it personally, you do not understand him. He is not mad at you; he is mad about the food. If you want him to go away … do it right."

I smiled when he told me this. I told him that he hit the nail on the head. I will always tell my cooks when the food is not right. I will just as quickly tell them when the food *is* right. This is actually my favorite part of being a chef. I love to look at my cooks' food and see that it is perfectly cooked, well seasoned, and well presented. I make a point to let the entire staff know what a good job this or that person did. It is another time when I get to see that twinkle in their eyes. I see how proud they are about doing it right. It makes it all worth it.

The payoff with my management style is that many of my employees have grown to be very good culinarians. I have seen many get promoted to directors, regional chefs, supervisors, and managers. I have seen that twinkle in their eye when they produce a good meal. The amazing thing is that the twinkle did not exist before. They never had anyone encourage them to grow, allow them to be wrong, and teach them how to correct their mistakes. They never had anyone who held them to high standards and wouldn't let up on quality. The old term that the cream always rises to the top is true. I like to believe that I have made a difference in people's lives. There are some who would disagree with this, but those would be the ones who never cared about the food they served and were let go. Like I always say, "You want to cook bad food, go work for the competition.

My most memorable moment was when I went to a large catering event at UNC Hospitals. I was reunited with my old cooks, whom I had not seen for many months. It was good to get reacquainted with them. One of the cooks who I truly thought would not make it was there. He was a talented cook but had a lot of issues. He saw me and he came up and said, "I made Black Hat Level One." He had his jacket on with his name embroidered on it and the title of Black Hat Chef. I was so proud of him. The chef I saw before me was a different person than the hospital cook I'd seen a year ago. He had grown to understand that what we were trying to do was not an impossible task. It was not unreachable. It was really quite easy: treat the food with respect, and you will get a good product. I was so happy that the people at UNCH made my Black Hat Chef program become such a success. It is all I ever wanted.

I often tell my employees that poor patient satisfaction is easy. Having a high patient satisfaction perception takes an enormous amount of work. It is not a race—when you cross the line, you have not won; you have to keep working to hold your position. You cannot stop there.

When we first hit 90 percent, we celebrated. This meant that, in our third-party survey that went to actual patients who had been discharged, we were at the top 10 percent of the country. We had made it. We were on top of the world! I told my staff, "Getting here was hard, but staying here will even be harder."

You can never stop, never have a bad day, and always strive to the next level. *You must constantly inspect what you expect.* You must sit for hours on the line watching how the food is prepared, follow your people who deliver the trays, hold everyone accountable, be fair, be firm, and celebrate your success. The most important thing is you must connect with the patients. Do these things and you will be successful.

The story at Rex is a story of victory. We took over from a multi-billion-dollar company. We had little money, poor equipment, and an untrained staff. However, we had a vision of what we wanted. We achieved what we wanted through hard work, a dedicated management team, and an awesome staff. They rose to the challenge.

To be successful in this business, you must always look for ways to improve. This is something I always do. I am always pushing for more, sometime at the behest of my staff. They always say that I can never sit still. I am always looking for the next great idea. They are right. I live in a world of constant change.

I recently told my executive chef that the ninetieth percentile is for wimps. I want to be at the 100 percent. He looked at me and said, "Great, I am going to have a stroke." However, the truth is that I am so very proud that we are at the top of our game, and people like my chef Ray D'Ottavio are the ones that make it happen.

The Patient

The patient says, "Doc, it hurts when I do this ....".
Then don't do that.

—Henny Youngman

I've spent most of this book talking to cooks and chefs and directors of food services. But since patients are key players in the hospital system, whether they realize it or not, let me take this chapter to address patients directly. You are the reason we are here—don't let us forget it.

As the patient, you are the reason why we are all here. Our job is to take care of you. When it comes to getting the food you want, all you have to do is ask. The first thing you should do is ask your doctor what diet you are on. The doctor is the one who prescribes it, not the food people. We just do what is told to us. We cannot make changes without a doctors approval. Make sure you understand what that diet means. If the doctor is unable to explain it correctly, ask for a dietitian to help.

The dietitian will explain your diet in full. He or she will tell you what you can and cannot eat—the medical condition you are in may be the result of or affected by the foods you are eating—and it is a great chance to get free advice on your diet. You are already spending a lot of money in your hospital stay. Take advantage of the fact that there is a team of people who understand how food interacts with the body and can help you make good choices.

The most important thing you can do is order your own food. If they try to send you a "Chef Special," ask your nurse what that meal is. It could very well be something you absolutely do not want to eat. The result will be that you will have to wait for an edible meal for a very long time. Make sure that you ask questions about what is available, considering your diet.

Be specific about what you want served with your food. Remember, the mentality of most hospital food services is if you do not ask for it, you will not get it. If you want creamer for your coffee, ask for it. If you want skim milk with your coffee, just ask. We have patients who want a latte from our Starbucks operation, and if they ask, we get it for them. If you want syrup with your pancakes, guess what, if you don't ask, you may not get it. You are the customer; if you ask, you will receive—but you have to ask.

If you do not get what you want, ask for the director of Food and Nutrition. He or she has the motivation to make you happy. There are bonuses in jeopardy—I kid you not; patient satisfaction is a key driver in management bonuses. Their very jobs are sometimes in question, so these are the people you need to speak to first. Do not ever leave the hospital mad at the food service staff. They will always try to make things better. Get what you want Be the squeaky wheel. We are here for you and will do whatever we can to make your stay as pleasant as possible.

The Hospital Food Service Worker

You never really understand a person until you consider things from his point of view.

—Harper Lee
Atticus's advice to his daughter, Scout, in *To Kill a Mockingbird.*

First, please remember why you are there. We are paid to provide some form of comfort to our patients, visitors, and fellow staff members. I can't tell you how many family members I have seen crying and upset about the news they have received. One such incident occurred when I was in DC. I vividly remember a family of about eight people hugging and crying together. Their ages ranged from about eight to over eighty years old. I asked a nurse who was helping them what was going on and if there were any way I could help. She told me that they had taken the grandmother off life support—the matriarch of the family had died. I approached the family and asked if I could get them a private room with some hot coffee and food. They were so relieved—I could see that they were in desperate need of some privacy and just wanted to get away.

I managed to get a small conference room for them, and my staff brought them coffee, sandwiches, and drinks. These people had been at Grandmother's bedside for so long, many had not eaten in twelve hours. The simple comfort of having some food and someone showing compassion went a long way. These are the reasons you are here.

Death, I suppose, is a sad part of life. It is how we respond to those who are suffering that makes us better people. I recently lost my dog—who could never be compared to someone's grandmother, but he was my best friend for twelve years and was extraordinarily special to me. The one incident that lifted me out of my grief was when my friends took me out for beers and were there for me. My managers also bought me a tree in his honor. I planted it and I look at it everyday. It meant so much and made his passing more bearable.

Little things make a difference, and the little things we food service workers can do to help our customers and our patients makes our jobs special. Remember every day you go to work, you can make a difference in someone's life. There is not a more honorable calling than that.

We must always remember that a hospital is not a place that people want to be. It almost always brings pain to not only the patient, but to the people who are visiting—the family and friends who care about their loved one.

There are horrible injuries, especially at level-one trauma centers. There is disease and death. I remember that when I was in Washington, DC my client had a picture of the hospital's medevac helicopter flying over the burning Pentagon after the attacks on September 11, 2001. It was a powerful picture of how much despair emergency responders and healthcare workers deal with every day.

Our hospital was a major receiving hospital for that attack. The employees were locked down, which was probably a good thing as the Metro and all roads in and out of DC were shut down. I spoke with many of the employees who were there that day, and they were proud of the fact that they had helped during our country's most desperate hour. We must allow the thought that however bad 9/11 was, many of our patients' family members are having their own personal 9/11 when someone dear to them is hurt or dying.

My wife works with cancer patients, and her stories are heartbreaking. We are all vulnerable, and all of the things we see and hear on a daily basis can happen to us or someone we love. If you are working in one state and your parents are in another, and God-forbid something happens to them and they end up in a hospital, wouldn't you want someone to go out of his way to treat them as a special patient, to treat them like family? I think about this all the time. I would want someone to treat my mother or father as their own family. Every day you go to work, you have the opportunity to do this. It is the greatest gift you can give someone who is desperately upset. So please do this; be the one who makes a difference.

The only thing that you can actually perceive as a happy moment in a hospital is when a woman gives birth to a healthy child. I used to work in a hospital that sent celebratory meals to new moms. This was a meal that was special. It was a choice of lobster tail or beef tenderloin. It was for the mom and dad to celebrate the birth of their child. I remember one particular incident when we got the order from a patient in the morning, and we sent it up at dinner. What we did not know was that the child had died during the day. Can you imagine the grief we caused by sending a celebratory meal to a mom who had just lost her baby? We have since fixed this, and I vowed to never let this happen again. It was awful—for all involved, believe me.

There are also many other happy moments that occur. There are incredible life-saving surgeries that happen every day. There are cancer patients who find their illness is in remission. There are skilled nurses and doctors doing whatever they can to heal people. Do not ever forget that you play a part in the healing process. Good nutrition is vital to better health, and nutrition is what we do.

The only other thing I can say about this is that we must learn to leave problems at the door. When delivering food to a patient, remember they are the ones in the bed, not you. I am sure that whatever problem we may have in our lives, it is not as big as theirs is today. We must always be courteous and kind and do what we are paid to do. Our job is to bring comfort to someone who needs comfort the most. If you feel that you are unable to provide compassionate service to someone in need, please get out of this business and go work somewhere else. What we do is not for everyone.

The Hospital Café and Its Visitors

There is no love sincerer than the love of food.

—George Bernard Shaw

The café should be an oasis to the madness that occurs in a hospital. Even though you work in the café and do not have direct patient care, it does not mean that you do not have influence on patient satisfaction.

Where do you think families of patients go to get away for a while? They come to see us. They may be happy their son was just saved in surgery from a car-crash injury or that the new prognosis was good for the treatment of cancer. These are happy things, relatively speaking, but the people coming through your lines may also be people who just learned that their loved one is not doing well, or that the surgery did not go as planned. They are having the worst day of their lives. They are upset and on edge; any little thing could set them off. Our job is to set them *at ease.*

We need to be the shelter in the storm. Our cafés should be warm and inviting. Our customers should feel like it is a comforting place to be. The food needs to be the best it can be, the coffee fresh, and we need to serve with a smile. Anyone not doing this is letting down the very people who need us most.

This also applies to our co-workers—the nursing staff, docs, and technicians who deal with grief and fear, pain and sadness all day long. They see people who are near the end of life or are very injured or sick. This must have an effect on the emotions of the caregiver. I know my wife has come home very upset when a patient has died or someone who they thought was going to be okay took a turn for the worse. We must remember their side of the story and be understanding of their needs. Give them a break!

However, there is another side to feeding our co-workers. Over the years of doing this, I have come to the realization that food service people are often the "door mats," that many think they can wipe their feet on and kick around.

Of course, we have to be the better person and turn the other cheek, smile, and try to kill them with kindness. This is harder for some than others. The poor cashiers are usually the ones who take the most grief.

Sometimes we deserve it. We often do not provide the service we should be providing. Sometimes the food is not as it should be, and often times the lines are long and people have to wait. This, of course, is not what we want in our operations, and we work hard to correct these things. However, most often we provide restaurant-quality food and service. Our customer service is often the best in the hospital. Even with all that we do to ensure great service, some people are downright mean to us.

Fellow employees can be especially brutal. They often take their frustration out on us and are quick to be critical. It is as if we are a lower class of people. Some of these folks should remember that they live in glass houses and should not throw stones—we are all here trying to accomplish the same mission.

I have seen bad service from many other areas in the hospital go unquestioned. One reason we get hit is that we sell food and everyone has an opinion about food. Most people do not have an opinion about medication or medical treatment, so they just go along with it. The other is we work in a giant fishbowl that everyone, at one time during the day, visits to receive our services.

Here is a true-life example of what I went through at a "hospital near you." This facility was providing a free throat clinic to test for cancer or other throat-related issues for employees. At forty years of age, I decided that maybe I should go. It could not hurt to have a look-see.

I went to the clinic and walked up to a counter that had two women sitting side by side. I approached the counter and stood there for almost three minutes before they even noticed me standing there, right in front of them. I could have touched them I was so close. The two women were having a conversation about one of their kids and were completely oblivious to me.

Finally, after I made many fidgety sounds—rattling keys, tapping my finger, coughing, etc.—one of them looked up at me and said, "Can I help you?"

I said yes and told them I was there for the free throat clinic that was being offered to employees. The lady shot me a disgusted look and said, "You have to wait in the other line." She then explained, "I handle the *actual* patients in this clinic and this clinic only." She pointed up. "Can't you read the sign"? I looked up and saw a sign above her reading, "Patient Admissions." I said, "Well … where do I go?" She then pointed to the sign above the lady sitting next to her and said, "You have to wait in *that* line."

I then took one step to the left and resumed waiting while the two continued talking. Several minutes went by with me standing there looking like a complete idiot, before the second woman actually said the words, "Can I help you?"

I was so stunned I almost fell over. Now, I am not known as a patient person, and they sure tried me that day. I said to her, "Now, I know you just heard the conversation I had with the lady sitting right next to you! What is it that you think I need help with?" She rolled her eyes and said that the employee screening was taking place at one o'clock and it is only twelve thirty, so I would have to wait. I was so disgusted I left and never had the screening.

If Food Services had ever done anything even remotely close to this incredible display of poor service, we would have had people sharpening their pitchforks and lighting their torches. It would never be allowed. Why is it allowed in other areas of the hospital? It occurs daily, and every co-worker who comes through our cafés should think about how they treat people.

The two people who were working that day at that clinic are not the norm. They are just the ones who should not be there. They should be let go to work in a convenience store. They would fit right in with the person talking on their cell phone. My old saying is *Pick a door, any door, and walk out, and don't come back.*

Food and Nutrition employees are often paid the lowest in a hospital setting. They work hard and try their best to do the job for which they were hired. These employees have been some of the hardest working people I have ever met. They deserve a break. However we are not perfect. If we do not provide the level of service that we should be providing, please tell us and we will correct it. I truly believe that there is no food service manager in the country that will not try to make things right. Most of my peers take their jobs very seriously and love what they do.

Hospital Administration and Its Contractors

The leader can never close the gap between himself and the group. If he does, he is no longer what he must be. He must walk a tightrope between the consent he must win and the control he must exert.

—Vince Lombardi

When I was working in Washington, I was asked to take our new hospital president to the doctor's lounge on the ground floor. He did not know the way and wanted an escort, someone who could explain what we did and how the operations worked. I met him in our café, and we walked down to the lounge. Halfway there, we were both approached by a visitor who was visibly upset. He said that he was trying to call his mother in DC to let her know how her daughter was doing. What he didn't know is that the phones in the hallway were for in-house use only and had no access to outside lines. He said he had gotten grief from the operator who would not help him or direct him to someone who could.

He asked us both, "Do you guys work here?" The president said, "Yes we do, and I am the president of the hospital and how can I help you?" The guy started to explain his story. When he told us that he was trying to get in touch with his family and had such trouble doing so, the president took out his own cell phone, handed it to him, and allowed him to use it. The guy called whomever he needed to speak to, handed back the president's phone, and thanked him.

The president asked his name and the name of the patient and apologized that he had had such a hard time. He didn't just ask, he wrote the name down on his notepad. He then handed his business card to him and said, "If you have *any* other problems while you are in this hospital, you call me personally." The thing that struck me was he really meant it. He was sincerely concerned about this person, a person he did not even know. It made an impression on me.

The guy said, "Well I guess I ran into the right person!" After he left, the president got on the phone and told someone that he wanted to speak to the Director of Communication and that he wanted that operator in his office. He then told me that we needed to make sure that the food to this patient was perfect and if we could do anything for their family, we should. I took this as not *if* we should, but rather *we better do this.* I am sure that he had a very enlightening conversation with that employee and her manager.

This was my very first interaction with anyone from hospital administration, much less the president. He was impressive, a guy who got things done. I could see why the hospital hired him. He was going to take this place to a new level. However, I knew the employees better than he did, and my first thought was, *you have a big job ahead of you.*

Sure, there were plenty of us who felt the same way he did, but there were plenty more who did not, and that was what was going to make it hard for him. I left him at the lounge and thanked him and wished him well. I hope that he did raise the level of satisfaction at that hospital. I left it soon after that encounter, so I do not know how things panned out, but if anyone could do it, he could.

Hospital administrations deal with so many problems that they make my job look easy. In today's financial situation, being responsible for the finances of a hospital and all that goes into it must be a daunting task. Their jobs are surely easier when all the departments in the hospital are doing what they are supposed to be doing, staying fiscally responsible, and extending the best care possible. It is one thing to have a visionary goal, to be financially sound, and to help develop the hospital into a cutting-edge medical center, but it is a far harder challenge to change the entrenched culture of the people working there.

In a hospital setting, there are many contractors who work in and around the hospital. There are information management companies, environmental services companies, security companies, medical equipment repair companies, linen companies, grounds keeping, and many more. It is impossible for a hospital to not have these contractors working every day, just to keep the institution going. It is a huge undertaking to run a hospital. One of the contractors that many hospitals employ runs their food service operations.

Food management companies number in the hundreds—there are many regional and small companies out there. The choices are endless, but the majority of the contract-held food service operations fall into one of the "big three" companies: Compass Group USA—with its health care division run by Morrison Management Specialists—Aramark, and Sodexo.

These companies are huge, and they all have many business segments. They operate higher-education accounts, the vast array of colleges throughout the country. They run health-care accounts that include hospitals, senior living centers, and nursing homes. They run sports venues such as football stadiums and arenas throughout the United States.

They also run what are called Business and Industry accounts. These usually comprise large companies, such as Google, that have employee cafeterias and event catering, and need someone to run it. This segment is actually where I started in contract management. I worked in the Bank of America building in downtown Phoenix, Arizona. These contractors also offer environmental services, linen services, and consulting. They do just about everything you could want.

The problem with these companies is that their loyalty is often in question. They are there to provide a service, but many times, it becomes more of a financial importance than a quality importance. I can say this because I have lived this for over sixteen years and was often caught in between the contractor and the client, company or institution. These contractors are, first and foremost, for-profit companies, and they will pursue that end by any means. I am not saying that making a profit is a bad thing; to be sure, it is an important part of their business model. What "for-profit" company would last very long if they did not make a profit?

However, working in that environment for so many years and having now worked in a self-operated world for the last four years, I see a distinct difference in how things are done. As a self-operated manager, I have loyalty to one company. It was so hard, especially as a director, working in a hospital as a contractor when I was caught in between what my company wanted and what the hospital wanted. Often, they had vastly different goals and objectives, and we had to balance the two and try to please everyone involved. It was pretty much a dog and pony show.

Things to Consider Before Engaging a Contractor

If you are a hospital executive and currently have a contractor or are thinking about it, consider these points and ask the hard questions to determine whether this is this the right choice.

- Are they tempting you by offering capital improvements up front?

If they say they will build you a new café, or put in room service, or maybe even build a new venue—remember that the patient day-rate they charge you will be higher in order to get that money back.

Keep in mind that if you decide at some point in time that you made the wrong choice, you will have to pay that money back before you can remove them.

Let me discuss some of the strategies that are used. I believe that most operators in all three companies are of the highest moral standards. They do not get as big as they are by ripping off their clients. They build relationships and offer a product that, quite frankly, many self-operated hospital food-service operations cannot provide. However, it is still a game, and if you know how the rules are played, you have a better chance at winning.

- How do they affect your patient satisfaction scores?

This is the benchmark against which you can hold contractors accountable, and it is easily measured. As the administrator, you must make this goal reasonable and attainable. Having an expectation of patient satisfaction from your contractor that is higher than from other departments is unrealistic and detrimental toward their success. Keep the expectations at a fair level of play. However, many contracts have financial penalties for not reaching these goals. Make sure that this is in your contact and hold them accountable for their scores. These scores are the best way to measure how they are participating in bringing your hospital to a level of excellence.

If they are not doing what is expected, make sure you exercise this penalty. There is no better way to get their attention than to take money from them. This single act will send warning bells throughout the hierarchy of the company. They are so worried about client-retention that they will act swiftly to address it. I have seen teams of people come from all over the country to fix a problem. If they know that they are being held accountable, they will do the best job they can.

One senior manager of a company I was working for told me to never bring this clause up to the hospital clients. This, of course, was when our scores were low, and no one was all that concerned about what the patients were saying; rather they were worried about the financial penalty. Check the fine print and work with your contractor to ensure that patient satisfaction is the highest concern.

- How will you be charged and what savings will be passed on to you from your contractor's *purchasing power*?

Find out what you are being charged for your floor stock and where it is going. Floor stock refers to the supplies we bring up to the nursing stations that patients might need throughout the day. Things like sodas, milk, juices, crackers, peanut better, jelly, snacks, etc.

Every hospital has different inventories that they carry. These items are also the most abused items that have ever graced a hospital. I think that probably only half of what is sent to the floors is actually consumed by patients. Every nurse, doctor, environmental service worker, nursing assistant, or whoever is walking by has access to these items. Why buy soda when you get one for free? You all know this happens, and we know it too. The biggest culprit is the coffee. If you ever want to save a lot of money, look into how much free coffee goes out the door. Much of this is going to your staff. If this is what you want, then it is a good satisfier. If you did not, then you may want to check it out. Have the nurse-managers put it in their budgets; you will see the abuse quickly curbed when they are held accountable.

Most floor stocks that contractors supply are a pass-through cost. This cost is called *out-of-rate*. The contractor's bill is cost-based on patient days. This is for the food that goes to the patient for regular meals. Anything outside this rate, like floor stock, doctor lounges, catering, and nourishments are out-of-rate costs and are billed separately.

What happens in most hospitals with contractors is that the client receives a bill every month. In this bill are the costs for patient days and all ancillary costs, including floor stock. First thing to do is ask for back-up documentation of every floor that received floor stock. Look at these numbers and if anything seems out of the ordinary, meet with that unit manager and make sure that these numbers are correct.

A good example would be a high charge for coffee on a pediatric floor. I have seen this over and over. The kids on that floor are not drinking the coffee—it is the kid's parents and the staff.

If this is what you want to drive satisfaction, then allow it, but just be aware of where your money is going. Insist that they have signed receipts from someone on the floor proving these goods have been received. If any floor stock bill is submitted without a signature, do not pay it. This will ensure that someone is checking that the food has been delivered. I can assure you that when they get the food from their vendors, they have someone checking it to ensure they are getting what they pay for. Remember, they pay the food invoices, so it is important to them. This is your invoice; it should be important to you.

Ask frequently to audit prices against what they charge. Ask to see an invoice from their prime distributor. They will balk and say that their pricing is proprietary, but remember back to the day they did their sales presentation. One of the things they most definitely talked about was their purchasing power. They told you that by having them come on board as a contractor, they could save you lots of money. They have their own purchasing arm of the company that can make nationwide deals to save you money. Remember that? Tell them that if you are being charged a pass-through cost, you should have the right to see that cost.

I recently took over operations from a contractor and managed to acquire a few of their invoices—my costs were actually cheaper than theirs. This is due to the fact that we belong to a group purchasing organization; we get the same benefits of purchasing power that they claim to own. There are also many rebates that come back from distributors, which as a contract-managed account you will never see. As a self-operated food service, you reap the awards of these programs, which can add up into thousands of dollars coming back to your hospital, rather than their corporate offices. If there is low-hanging fruit available from vendor relationships, it should be yours. Even though contractors pay the invoices for food, you pay for their costs through the patient day-rate. They get the rebates, but bill you for the true value of the food. I bet they do not back out the rebates. Ask the questions—better yet, ask for the rebates. See what they say about that. It's your money; if they do not give you the rebate in cash, they should use it to credit your patient day-rate.

Note any additional fees and costs listed on the contractors' invoices. At least one of the big three contractors will likely post a one percent additional charge for *handling and invoice processing.* If this is in your contract, that is okay, but I urge all administrators to look at this cost very closely. This is a junkyard charge, and it can add up to thousands of dollars per year. Think about it—they buy the food, which you pay for; then they receive the rebates and the profits from selling food in your hospital, and final insult, they have the nerve to turn around and charge you a percentage of all your costs to process the invoices that they bill you with. Whoever got that idea past the client probably got a raise and a dinner out on the town.

- How much are you paying for the corporate and regional chefs, and where will they be when you need them?

The contractors' top chefs tend to only show up when there are problems or when there's a new retail program to push, which by the way, makes them money. But look closely into your bill—you may find that you are being charged overhead for their salaries. I know when I was in the contractor world, I paid a portion of their salaries, yet I never saw them.

Bottom line, if you pay monthly, you should see them monthly. Insist that you meet with them monthly, and ask what they are doing to provide better food to your patients—get them involved. Many of the chefs I have encountered are more than willing to help, once they get in front of the client—unfortunately, you might have to ask. Get their cell phone numbers, and get in touch with them any time you have problems with the food. That is what they get paid for. Most important, get your chef and the director in your office together to formulate a plan that will get you to where you want to be. Pass that on to the corporate chef to implement at that level; do not expect them to know what you want. You have to meet regularly and discuss your vision.

The most important question that you can ask them is what they are doing to improve patient food. Do not get caught up with the retail operations. These may get you great accolades from the staff, but patient satisfaction is where the rubber meets the road. Ask them how they are going to implement a training program. Ask them what they are going to do to bring your food to the next level. Many times the local management is not capable of doing this. You hired a company, not just the local management team: make sure you tap into all of their assets. They have a lot, and much of it could help you drive your program. If they are not doing this, call them out on it.

- How are profits split in your contracts?

A Profit Split clause is often in contracts to help keep the contractors from making too much profit at your hospital; this is when you reach a predetermined sales figure, over which the profits are split. The reason this exists speaks to my point that most of their effort goes to retail sales. The contractor will subtract their additional costs from sales over that limit, and then split the profit with the hospital.

Here is an example: Your agreement limits the contractor's sole profits to $1 million in sales; if there is anything over that in sales, the profit would be split.

So, let's say you had $1.2M in sales:

That's $200,000 sales dollars over the contract limit. Subtract from that $154,000 in total costs for that portion of the sales. (The contractor reports $90,000 in food costs (determined at 45 percent of total food costs), $14,000 in paper costs, and $50,000 for all other fixed and non-controllable costs).

That leaves $46,000 in split-profits, which when divided by two, gives $23,000 to the hospital and $23,000 to the contractor.

What I have learned over the years is that there is no way for the contractor to know what their food and paper costs are in retail operations alone. Every hospital I have been at orders food and paper from their distributors for the entire operation—retail and patient feeding. The two sides of the business are not separated out. The true food cost can only be determined by knowing exactly what food dollars were spent on retail and what was spent on patient feeding. They just do not know this. So how do they know to charge 45 percent of food costs in their profit and loss statement (P&L) to determine how much you will receive? The answer is that this is a made up number. If they are trying to displace food cost in a contract like this, they will dump cost into retail which, in turn, reduces the amount they have to reimburse.

They will come up with a million reasons why this is untrue. They will do everything to not divulge this information. My point is simple: this is your money, and you have the right to know where these figures came from. You would certainly ask when renegotiating a contract with an insurance or medical-supply company.

Have them run a potential food cost estimate on their retail operations. This is a sales-mix analysis of what is sold and how much is sold. You simply take the cost of every item sold (which any good operator will have) and multiply it by the amount sold in, say, a two-week period. As all food sold has a different food cost, this will give an average, or *mix* of the cost. Take the total cost and divide it by the total sales for that period, and you will have a potential food cost. Now, you do have to have some wiggle room, say 2 percent. This will take into consideration employee meals, waste, food that was returned, fryer oil, burnt food, food dropped on the floor, etc. Any situation where they would have lost some of the food without generating sales should be considered a cost and included in that figure.

Use *this* new number to decide what the food cost assigned to retail is. Wait till you see their faces when you tell them this is how you will determine the figures! Do the same with paper and look closely at all other costs. I assure you that there is money that is rightfully yours that they are keeping. I am sure retail costs do not come near 45 percent.

If you are having doubt on the validity of the amounts you are being charged, call the vice president of the contract company you have hired. Do not talk only to the director or the general managers. Bring them into the loop, but do not settle for their word or even the word of the district manager. These companies are very honest at the corporate level and, for the most part, at the unit level. I have worked with some very ethical people who would never do anything dishonest in any way to deceive the client.

Nonetheless, I have seen some shady deals go down. I will tell you that most of the dishonest things I have seen are due to the intense pressure these directors are under. They know if they submit bad weekly numbers, there will be hell to pay. The people who write these contracts often know that the goals are unattainable. The thought is if they put what it would really cost to run the operation in the contract, they will lose it to an underbidding competitor. What these sales people and VPs think is that once they get the contract, they can renegotiate it later. Get in the door—that is what is important.

The problem is that the director who first gets the account has such a hard time making the numbers that were set that he panics when he see the costs for the week not where they should be. He knows that his boss is going to be very upset, and that is where honest people become dishonest.

I have seen reputable directors fudge the numbers on their inventory just to make the food cost what it is supposed to be. This is a slippery slope and only leads to continued false numbers, and ultimately, to poor food and poor service.

I once had a purchasing manager come to me and say that she had turned in her inventory to the director and he was very mad at her. He had run the numbers, and his food cost was not where he wanted it to be. He actually wrote a number on a piece of paper and said, "This is what your inventory needs to be." It was a fabricated number, and she was caught in the middle of a huge lie and, possibly, something that could get them both fired. This kind of stuff happens all the time.

These directors will be forced to cut costs in the food they buy. Now, they do work off a managed order guide and are not allowed to just buy whatever they want, but they also take short cuts. The food that you saw from the corporate chefs that came during their sales pitch, well cooked and well presented, may not be what your staff is eating in the cafés. It will most certainly not be what your patients are eating.

It will be a much more conservative form of food. I once saw contractors in hospitals using a ground-beef mixture. This mixture had potato starch and other fillers mixed in the ground beef to make it cheaper. They were not using 100 percent ground beef. This should not be allowed. It was never allowed when I worked for that management company, and I was puzzled at how they were buying it. They also looked at many other ways to cut their costs in the food. They did not, for the most part, look at ways to streamline production or the way they were doing business. They would rather look at the client—and ask for money.

I actually saw a contractor (one of the big three) go to the client and tell him that they had missed their sales projection, and as a result, needed to increase the patient day-rate to make up the loss of revenue. Unreal! Retail revenue is their responsibility. They are the ones who control that. If they had cooked good food, done some marketing, and worked as a team to drive sales, they would have met their sales goal. They chose to be lazy and produce substandard food, with the result that customers went somewhere else to eat.

It was their fault. How could they even suggest that it was their client's responsibility to fill in that gap? They wrote the contract; they projected their own sales. Shame on them for not doing what they said they were going to do. I have been in places where we have increased sales by 50 percent in the first six months. You have to work hard to get these results. Sitting on your butt and serving bad food is not going to do it.

My suggestion is that you fully understand the contract and hold them to each and every piece of it. Make sure that you use all the assets that you are paying for. If they move a manager or someone leaves, make sure they replace that person or that they reduce the patient day-rate. The salaries of these people are in that rate. I cannot stress it enough: get what you are paying for.

Make sure they are providing the best food and service possible. They are all capable of it. They have thousands of extremely talented people working for them, and they are able to do it. They just sometimes get complacent, as we all do, and they need a little nudge now and again.

Most importantly, eat the food. You are the best judge of what is good and what is not. If it is not good, make them fix it.

Nursing Homes

Life's tragedy is that we get old too soon and wise too late.

—Ben Franklin

Along with my duties at the main hospital at Rex, I also have the responsibility of providing food service for two separate nursing homes. These homes both have their own kitchens and staff. The food is very different from what we serve in the main hospital. It was a challenge for me to say the least. I had never worked in this environment before and no idea what I was in for.

Nursing homes and other long-term-care facilities are the last stop for many of our patients. They are also temporary places for people who are recovering from strokes or surgeries and need rehabilitation to get their lives back in order. They are often very sad places, and it makes it even more important for us to do our jobs.

The people who work in these homes are some of the most dedicated people I have ever met. They go out of their way everyday to make the last few weeks, months, or even years of those they care for the best that they can be. The level of care that the residents in our nursing homes receive is probably the best in the country. I am proud to be associated with these folks. I am, however, not proud of the food. It is not like anything you would imagine. That's why we have begun a yearlong journey to make this food better. We want our food services to be, in addition to the great medical care our residents receive, the very reason they choose to come to us.

We have people who are too old and sick to care for themselves. Our job is to provide a service that they can no longer do. It really is an important job. Someday we will be there. I have always believed in Karma—what goes around comes around—so we better take care of our elderly. They are the ones that shaped our generation, and we owe it to them. If we don't, how can we expect to be cared for when we are in their place?

When I walk through these homes, I see grandmothers and grandfathers. These folks have cooked their whole lives; they know what they like and how food should be cooked. They may not be chefs, but they know how a Thanksgiving turkey should taste. They know what a good soup is, and they certainly know how they like their vegetables cooked. They are more opinionated than our acute care patients in the main hospital—after all, this is where they live now; they want it to feel *and taste* like home. They are dependent on us to give it to them.

So, what are they eating? The challenge with older patients is their inability to eat the way the way they used to. They often have problems with their teeth; they may have had a stroke and become unable to chew food as a healthier person would; their digestive systems may have broken down. Life is harsh, growing old is a fact of life and it is not always pretty. The food that we serve has to be modified in order for many elderly patients to eat it. In other words, there is a lot of pureed food being served.

As a chef, this has been the hardest thing for me to overcome. Seeing pureed food quite frankly makes me sick to my stomach. In order to understand this type of food, I had to understand the residents who were eating it. I spent a lot of time talking to them and asking them what they liked and disliked. I found out that they disliked spicy foods and liked their vegetables cooked to death.

I studied the food in depth and saw that it was shameful on every level imaginable. It was wrong. It was really wrong.

The Cooks

The cooks who work in nursing homes are, for the most part, good, hardworking people. They do try, but they have absolutely no idea what good food is. The rampant problem in this side of the industry is that no time or energy has ever gone into training these folks on how food should be cooked.

It is not their fault. They were probably once a tray line employee some twenty years ago, and then they moved into a cook's position, shown a few shortcuts, and then promoted to *the* Cook. That was the extent of their culinary training.

Cooks get paid more, so it is lucrative for a long-time food-service worker to want to be a cook. Many of these folks should have never been asked to be a cook, but some manager, at sometime, thought it was a good idea. The result is that you have poorly prepared food by people who fall into a routine of bad production practices and are never taught how to be a proper culinarian. In fact, most of them do not even aspire to be that. They just do their "8" and go home.

It is very difficult for me to come into these places and be overly critical. It really is not fair to them. It is all they know, and they see nothing wrong with what they are doing.

I believe the biggest problem is management. They allowed—and continue to allow—this to happen, and I am not sure why. It could very well be that they feel they do not have money in the budget to provide good food. This is complete nonsense, as cooking food correctly does not cost any more money than cooking it badly. It actually could cost less. The other reason could be that they just do not know any better. A combination of these factors ultimately leads to bad food.

I was once asked to speak to a group of nursing home managers at their annual convention. Angelo and I drove up to Washington, DC and met the group of about 150 people. Our speech was about the "Black Hat Chefs" and how we, as an industry, should be training our cooks to meet today's customer expectations. We talked about using fresh produce, locally farmed meats when possible, and most important, bringing restaurant-quality food to our patients and residents.

We talked about the necessity of well-executed food. I asked the group how many of their cooks used the steamer for everything possible. They all kind of chuckled. The cooks in this arena use that damn steamer for everything!

I told the group that I have actually seen a cook steam cubed beef, noodles, and then steam the gravy. Gives you a headache just trying to imagine it, doesn't it? This cook then mixed it all together and called it Beef Stroganoff. This is the type of cooking that everyone in the room was used to. It was completely acceptable in their eyes. "The rules say we have to feed the residents. No rule says it has to be restaurant quality." Well, I can tell you that the rule at Rex is that it *must* be restaurant quality or we do not serve it … *period!*

The entire time we were speaking, it was like we were speaking in an ancient tongue. They had no idea what we were saying. There was so little emotion in that room, it freaked me out. I asked the group if they had any questions, and not one person raised their hand. The worst vibe I got was that no one understood the importance of what we were saying; bad food would continue to be served, exactly what I had spent the last eight years fighting against.

The most horrific thing I have ever seen is how we handle pureed food. The rules that govern nursing homes are very strict; all facilities have to be inspected to ensure that the rules are being followed. These inspectors look at everything from cleanliness to how medications are dispensed, accessibility to medical treatment, and the quality of that treatment, as well as compliance regarding the food served to the residents. One of the many rules is that the people on pureed diets must be offered the same variety of food as those people on regular diets. This is a great rule, as I am sure that many of these people were fed horrible concoctions of who knows what, plopped on a plate.

At Rex, we do not do this. Our food is the same food that is served to our regular patients. The difference is that we puree it before we serve it. However, we could still do better.

I once went into one of our homes and saw something I could not, in my wildest dream, identify. It was a UFOP—Unidentified Food on Plate. I asked just what in the hell this was, and the person said it was a pureed pizza. I said, "What?" Not sure that I had heard her correctly, I asked again. She said that they had pizza on the menu and were told the pureed diets get the same meal, just pureed. I cannot even tell you what it looked like, other than the result of a wild night of drinking, ending up in a pizza joint, and then later getting sick. That is exactly what it looked like.

I met with my team and told them if we are to serve pureed food, we had to think about how the food looked when it was pureed. Pizza would certainly never be served like that again. If we were to serve pizza, why could we not puree the dough, top it with sauce, and then top it with cheese? We could make it look like a pizza, which would allow the resident to maintain some dignity.

Dignity—what a strong word that is. The people we are feeding are part of what Tom Brokaw calls the Greatest Generation. These men and women were the ones who fought in World War II, Korea and Vietnam. They were also the women who worked as "Rosie the Riveter" to help the war effort. This was a very important task, and without them, the outcome of the war may have been different. These people have families, had amazing lives that we could not even imagine. I met a guy with a

PhD in mathematics from Duke University who had worked for President Richard Nixon in the White House. He'd had a stroke, and the way he was trapped in his own body was very humbling to me. He was probably the smartest guy I ever spoke to, but the image of him was so much the opposite.

Younger people often look at older people with indifference. What a mistake that is. Our elders have so much to offer. They know more than we do. They have lived lives full of experiences, challenges, sadness, and joy. Their youth is still inside them, while our maturity has yet to match theirs. We should look at them as inspirations in how to run our lives. They have already done what we plan to do. They are entitled to even more than dignity; they are entitled to honor.

I have a theory that as we get older, we begin to see some sort of purpose in how things are supposed to be. I am in my mid-forties now, and I see things much differently from how I used to. I feel this is due to the experiences that I have gained over the years. I know that the things I have done in my life have molded me and made me who I am. I have seen and done a lot, but I have not seen the things that the residents of these homes have seen. They could teach us all a lesson on how the world works. I know that age brings wisdom, and these people are much older than me; therefore, they are likely to be much wiser.

I have had managers who were much younger than me who would frequently challenge me on my ideas. I do readily accept this, as often I am wrong, and their ideas are actually better—however, I have lived and experienced things that they have not. I often see ideas that are brought up by my managers that I have tried—years ago—and they did not work. On the other hand, they might bring up things that I never thought of. I tell my younger managers that when they were doing bong hits in college, I was running a business. So when I propose an idea, I usually have some experience to back it up. "Trust me," I tell them, "I know what I am doing. I have done this before." Sometimes they believe me; sometimes they don't. Sometimes I am right; sometimes I am wrong. But respect is a two-way street. It is no different with our elderly patient-residents.

The people we serve in these homes are some of the most interesting people I have ever met. I once saw a guy who had the insignia of the 82nd Airborne on his ball cap. I was of course drawn to him. We spoke for almost an hour. He had fought in the Hurtgen Forest during WWII. This was one of the bloodiest battles our country had ever fought. He was a war hero, and if anyone thought that I was going to do him the disservice of serving UFOP to him, they obviously did not know me very well. We were going to change this, and we were going to change this quickly.

We are in the midst of transforming the way our residents eat. We are putting interesting and exciting choices on the menu. We are designing a pureed menu that works. This is our biggest challenge, as pureed food is not always very attractive, but it needs to look halfway appetizing. The food will be molded to make it identifiable. If our residents are eating green beans, I want them to be able to look at it and know that it is green beans. Food is first perceived by the eyes. If it looks good, the brain processes it as good, and the taste will follow. The old saying, "You eat with your eyes," surely applies. This should be our standard. *The food needs to look good, and the people who eat this food deserve to eat it with dignity.*

Imagine having a stroke—or just getting old, as we all will, if we're lucky—and having to eat UFOP. To me, it would be like eating baby food. At eighty, ninety, a hundred years old, they are not babies. They are grown men and women. They should not have to eat baby food. They are our parents and our grandparents. Start treating them that way. All too soon, they will be our brothers and sisters, our husbands and wives; they will be us.

We have a long way to go in this part of the industry, but I am assured that things will change, and I like to think that we are leading that change. I want our residents to be proud of the food we serve. I also want our employees to be well trained and to understand their true mission: serve great food. Maybe then, we can all be happy about getting old.

The World We Live In

No, you do not understand, this is not made up, it is for real. This is what we have to go through. In the course of your day, please ask yourself ... Do you have to deal with this nonsense, or is the biggest issue of your day pretty much relegated to what you are going to have for lunch?

—A Colleague

someone dear to me said this in one of our many conversations with employee relations with the SEIU looking on. For the first time in my life, I actually said, "You go girl"... Priceless! However, the conversation was still painful.

In the health care industry, we come across many insane and unbelievable things that occur every day in our kitchens—things that most people would not believe. I talk to many of my chef friends who work in high-class hotels and restaurants throughout the country, and they just do not believe the things we go through. They actually say to me, "You are making that up." I tell them that it is not made up—it is my reality.

These stories are the end to my book, but they make up "a day in the life" of what I go through. It is painful and unbearable at times, but for some strange reason, I have thrived in this world.

These things you just cannot make up ...

The Torn Bread Incident

We had an infusion center that served approximately forty people per day. Our job was to provide a sort of boxed lunch for the patients who had to go there for medical treatment. One day, I went through the kitchen to see what the cooks were doing and saw a sheet pan with sandwiches on it. I immediately noticed that the sandwiches were torn apart. I asked why these sandwiches looked like this. The employee told me that she could not find a knife, so she actually tore the sandwiches in half with her hands. These sandwiches looked like a horse had gotten to them; they were horribly mangled and actually had finger indentations in them. They were freakin' torn in half! Where have you ever seen that? Where have you ever even heard of that?

I was stunned and could not move for a few moments. As the realization of what had happened hit my brain, I just had to ask, "Why on earth would you do that?" She looked at me with complete indifference and said that she could not find a knife. I walked over to the prep area and found a knife within seconds. I asked her, "What about this knife?" She couldn't have cared less. We wrote her up, but the union fought it. We had sixteen hours of grievances over that one. We won in the end, but the very fact that we had to argue our case left me very sad. This person had not one bit of love for food in her body, and she was one of my cooks! Painful.

The One Boot Incident

I was working in my office, which faced the kitchen. I heard a strange sound coming down the hallway. It was a sound like "ca—clop, ca—clop." I looked up and I saw one of my cooks walking past my office. He had on one boot and one sneaker. He passed my office, and I was going to just let it go, but my curiosity got the best of me. I just had to find out. It was killing me to know. I got up and asked him why on earth he was wearing one boot and one sneaker.

His response was that he woke up and could not find his other sneaker. He said he had to get to work, so he just put one of each on. I was perplexed and amused by this. I asked him, "If you could not find your other sneaker, why did you just not wear your other boot? Why did you wear one of each?" He was so puzzled by my question. He stood there for a few minutes before responding, "I did not think of that." He was also one of my cooks … painful.

The Raw Chicken Incident

I went to one of our doctors' lounges to check on things. I passed our salad bar, which had about twenty-five ingredients in it. I noticed that the chicken was completely raw. It looked like it had been on the grill for maybe twenty seconds, just enough to get the outside cooked, but the inside was completely raw. I pulled it off the salad bar and brought it back to the kitchen. I approached the cook and asked her what the deal was. She said that she thought it was cooked and saw no reason for me to question her.

We counseled her for serving raw chicken on a salad bar, but of course, we were grieved by the union. They stated that she was not trained on the "proper cooking of chicken." In the grievance, I asked, "In the twenty-five years you have been a cook, you have not learned how to cook chicken? If I were the guy who vacuumed the car and did oil changes at Jiffy Lube for twenty-five years, I would probably know how to change the oil in a car. She was a cook for twenty-five years, and she served raw chicken? We spent hours on that one with the union, but we eventually won. Even the arbitrator could not believe her story. She was also one of my cooks. Painful!

The Scratchy Back Incident

I once saw a cook serving on our line who actually took his carving knife, pushed it under his chef coat, and scratched his back. This was done in front of the customers that were in his line. He took the tip of the knife and went under his chef coat and scratched his back with the knife. He then pulled the knife out and went to carve the meat. I stopped him in front of our horrified customers and had to explain to him why he was wrong. He of course did not get it. He was also one of my cooks. Oh, this is so *painful!*

The Raw Pie Incident

I once went to an event at one of our college campuses. They were putting on an event for the public opening of one of their new schools. Our job was to provide the food for the reception. They had a full menu, including carved meats, salads, and dessert. The desserts they had that day were apple pies.

I walked in about a half hour before the event. I walked up and down the buffet lines as the workers were scurrying around finishing last minute details. I stopped in front of the dessert station and looked at the pies. Something was not right. They looked really pale. I then realized that the pies were raw. Someone had taken the pies out of the box, cut them into pieces, and then plated them. They had no clue that the pies had not been baked.

I went to the manager and told her that the pies were not cooked. Just then, the people attending the reception started to come in the door. The look on her faces was that of sheer terror. She did not know what to do. I had a few people pull the pie plates off the line. Needless to say, our guests did not get apple pie that day. When I ask her who would do such a stupid thing, she replied that it was her lead cook who did it. She put out raw apple pies, and no one ever noticed. This was *her* cook … Painful.

The Gloves in the Bathroom Incident

I was working one day in our main kitchen. We had a men's bathroom just outside the kitchen. It was mostly used by our staff, but was available to the public. I went in and saw one of my cooks at the urinal. After he was done, he turned around, and I noticed that he was still wearing his food-prep handling gloves. These are gloves that we wear when handling ready-to-eat foods. They are supposed to be used for one task; then, you have to wash your hands and put on a new pair before beginning a new task. This guy was actually going to the bathroom while wearing his gloves. I could not believe it. I told him to take his gloves off and wash his hands.

He began to argue with me. He absolutely did not get what I was saying. All of our employees had food-safety training. He had that training but still did not care. We eventually fired that guy. I had never seen anything like this before; I truly thought it was an anomaly. I swore I would never see it again. I was wrong. A few years later, I saw it again. The employees we were working with, many of them just flat out did not care about the safety of the people we were serving. And yes, he was one of *my* cooks … Painful.

The Cookie Pan Incident

We were going through a renovation in our main café. The construction guys had put up a dust barrier around one of our cooking stations to do some work. One day, I went behind the curtain to see how the work was coming along. I noticed that a sheet pan of cookies was still behind the line. This area had been a bakery, and someone had left cookies behind. I asked an employee to go back there and throw away the cookies as they had dust all over them. She said no problem and went behind the curtain.

The next day I went back there and saw that the sheet pan was still there, but the cookies were gone. I asked her later why the pan was still there. Her reply was, "You did not ask me to get the pan, only the cookies." I was dumbfounded. But I learned a lot that day—I learned that you had to be very specific when assigning tasks to employees. She did exactly what I asked her to do. In my world, you have to explain exactly what you want done. It is a shame, but it is reality, and of course, she was one of my cooks. Painful.

The Moth in the Mouth Incident

I was working in Arizona and had this employee who always had an issue. He was very loud, and he always liked to argue. He was the person who always held court, always had something to say. He was definitely a talker. He never stopped. One day, he wanted to talk to me in private about some ridiculous issue he was having. We went outside, and he began to rant about something. As he was talking, a giant moth flew right into his mouth (this thing was the size of a small bird; it was huge). For the first time since I had known this guy, he stopped talking. He began to choke on this moth, hacking and spitting out pieces of it. It was the funniest thing I have ever seen. I was laughing so hard I could not breathe.

He finally got the moth out of his mouth, and I do not think that I will ever forget the look on his face. It was priceless. Between my laughter, I told him that it took a moth to shut him up. I had to sit down it was so funny. He had this look on his face … He had tears in his eyes from hacking. Man, it was something to see. He was completely silent.

As I am writing this, I am laughing just thinking about it. This was over sixteen years ago, but I remember it clearly. It was the funniest thing I have ever seen. After that day, he did not complain as much as he used to. I do think that moth was sent to shut him up. It was truly a memorable moment for me. Of course, he was one of my cooks … Very funny, but very painful.

The Seasoned Salt Incident

We were doing a big party for a college at which I was working. It was a full-service breakfast for four hundred people. We had set up various stations in our ballroom. We had an omelet station, carving station, and a huge buffet line.

Just before the meal started, I told one of my cooks to season the potatoes with our in-house seasoning blend. We used to make this in five-pound batches of salt, garlic, paprika, and other seasonings. We used it in many applications. I handed the cook the container that held the seasoning; it was probably eight pounds or more. I then went out to check the buffet. When I returned to the kitchen, I noticed that the container was empty. I panicked. I asked the cook, "Where did the seasoning go?" He said he put it on the potatoes. I ran out to the buffet and stopped the servers just in time. These potatoes had over eight pounds of salt on them!

I brought them back to the kitchen and asked the cook why he would do that. He said, "You told me to season them." I said, "I did not mean the whole container. Did you not think for even a moment that maybe this is a lot of seasoning?" He was a little embarrassed, and I think he got it. He actually turned out to be a very good employee. He went on to become a chef. I think he learned a lot from what he did and probably still talks about it today. It was painful, but could have been worse—that pan of potatoes could have been served!

The Drunken Interview Incident

I was interviewing an applicant for one of our retail operations. We met in the dining room, and I immediately smelled alcohol on his breath. I was just about to end the interview, when his wife showed up with three screaming kids. He began to talk to me about where he had worked. He was slurring his words and leaning forward with his head. He then yelled at his wife to "Shut those damn kids up!" I was appalled. He then began to yell at his wife, asking her what the name of his old supervisor was. She did not know, and they began to argue. He was calling her every name in the book. It got so bad I had to get up and call the campus police. They showed up and led the couple and their kids out the door. They were still yelling and cursing at each other as they were being escorted out.

I sat there in silence, reeling at what I had just witnessed. I then came up with some good tips for people interviewing for a job:

- Tip Number One: Never go to an interview drunk.
- Tip Number Two: Never bring your drunk spouse and kids to the interview.
- Tip Number Three: Never do anything that would lead the interviewer to call the police. This is really important; please pay attention to this one.

If any of these things happen, rest assured you will *not* get the job. This was extremely painful.

The Grease-in-the-Hair Incident

I was working at a university in Arizona. We had a full-scale bakery at this account. It was very well equipped and was a very busy place. We did our own donuts, breads, desserts, etc. It was really nice to have this operation. I have not seen anything of this scale since then. I was walking through our bakeshop one late afternoon. Most of the bakers had gone home, but there was one baker hanging around. I watched him take a gallon jug of canola oil and put it on the workbench. He then poured about a cup of it in a glass and then poured the oil on top of his head. He then rubbed the oil into his hair and shook the extra oil out.

He shook his head side-to-side, spraying oil all over the place. He then reached into his pocket and pulled out a comb and proceeded to comb his hair. He had it all slicked back. I was standing there in absolute amazement. I approached him and said, "Just what the hell are you doing?" He said he was greasing his hair. I pulled him into the office and explained that what he was doing was first and foremost the most ridiculous thing I have ever witnessed and the fact that he was doing this in a production kitchen was even worse. I made him clean up all the oil he had spilt. The amazing thing was that he did not think what he was doing was wrong and asked me why I was making such a big deal about it. He said he always greases his hair. I said, "Okay, *Bowser,* go grease your hair ... Just don't do it here." He was one of my bakers! Painful.

The Pulled-Over Catering Van Incident

We were catering a huge event on at the south end of campus. We had a box truck and a van filled with food heading toward the event. I left the kitchen a few minutes later and proceeded to drive across campus. I was waiting at a light and saw a police car fly by me. He had lights and sirens on and was in a big hurry. I went farther down the street and saw two police cars on the side of the road. They had pulled over our catering van. As I approached, they had my employee outside and spread-eagle against the van. They were in the process of handcuffing her when I pulled up and asked, "What is going on?" They told me she was wanted for dealing drugs, and they were taking her in. My first thought was, *What about the catering van?* It was packed full of our food for this catering event!

I had to wait around while they searched the van, but I finally got the food to the event. This caused our event to be late. It was hard to explain that one to the client … "Oh, sorry the event was late; one of our employees got busted on the way down here for selling drugs." It was unbelievable.

Needless to say, we fired her. It seems that while she was out doing catering events, she also had a side business selling weed out the back of our catering van. I had an event feeding five hundred people, and I had to deal with this nonsense. Painful!

The Bone-In Chicken Sandwich Incident

A patient had asked for a fried chicken sandwich. Someone on our line grabbed a sandwich bun and put a bone-in fried chicken breast on the bun, topped it, and sent it upstairs. The patient called down completely irate, rightfully so. He asked, "Who would do something so stupid? "How can I eat a sandwich full of bones?" Our patient-services manager apologized and said we would send another. Another sandwich was made—again with a bone-in fried chicken breast. I got the call in my office that this guy wanted to see a manager. I went upstairs and was at a complete loss of words. Not only did my staff do an unconceivable mistake by sending a chicken breast sandwich with bones in it, but we did it twice! *Unbelievable* would be an understatement.

I tried desperately to find out who did it, but I never did. I was going to make a sandwich for this person and say, "You eat it." I wanted to send this person to be studied. I wanted to know what made him tick. Who would do that? Even people who knew nothing about food would know not to do this. What was going through this person's mind when he grabbed a fried chicken breast with bones and slapped it on a bun? Very, very, very painful!

I could go on and on, but I will spare you the misery. I must say that even with all this, and how it seemed, at times, that my vision would never get to fruition, I have had some very good outcomes. I have worked in many places all around the country. I have met hundreds of people over the years. I have cooked for thousands of people and have always been appreciated by those I worked for.

I have met some incredible people. The good far outweigh the bad. Most of the people I have come across do care about what they do. It is a shame that we have to deal with the idiots of the world. In the end, my message is the same that I have always preached: *Serve Great Food.*

I hope that everyone who reads this book has a different opinion about hospital food. We are changing things for the better. It may take another five to six years to get the right people in place—those who care about food and about the people they serve.

I hope that the entitlement mentality will exit our business and that people will actually care more about the food they serve than what they think is due them. This is a stretch, but I believe someday it will be true.

I do not have the answers. All I can do is keep pushing my staff towards greatness. We can serve great food in this environment, the hospital environment. I prove it everyday. I end the book with this one thought:

In this business, we should always try to make a difference in someone's life. This may be as simple as a hot cup of coffee or a well-executed consommé. It may be a perfectly sautéed veal scaloppini or a well-dressed salad. It may be a duck confit that just melts in your mouth, or it may be a carne asada taco that makes you smile. It could be my beloved *mole* from Mexico or an incredible Cuban sandwich, *live from Miami Beach!* It may be perfectly cooked rice or a braised lamb shank. It could be a perfectly roasted top round of beef. It may even be the freshness of a handmade salsa or a perfectly roasted chicken with gravy made from the fond in the pan, not from a package.

It may be a hot meal served by people who care about what they do, served with a smile. Or, it may be the simplest thing we do—cook the food right and cook it as it was meant to be. Cook it like *you* care about what *you* do.

Whatever it is, if you are in the food business, serve your food with pride. Good food is good karma!

As the late Chef Papini, my old chef at the Culinary Institute of America used to say, "Cook it with love or do not cook it at all."

Postscript

I end this with a great big thank you to all the people who helped me over the years. I especially want to thank my current managers and friends who have made all this happen.

Going from 28 percent of our patients at Rex Healthcare saying we were excellent to, at the writing of this book, 94 percent, is not a solo accomplishment. It could have never been accomplished without the people who care as much as I do and try everyday they go to work to make things better. I mentioned these people at the beginning of the book, but they all deserve another mention:

Ryan Miller, Betsy Thomas, Ryan Conklin, Lyn Haft, Marlon Davis, Angelo Mojica, Chad Lefteris, Ray D'Ottavio, Cheryl D'Ottavio, Paul Berens, the guy with the moth in his mouth, and all the others who made this journey possible. Thank-you, and "here's to your health!"

—Jim McGrody

One more thing …

I wrote this book over a two–and-a–half-year span at my tiki bar—the bar my wife bought me and soon afterward regretted. Thank you, Alicia. I would never be where I am at without your love.

LaVergne, TN USA
16 February 2011
216751LV00002B/25/P